PENGUIN BOOKS

THE EXPERIENCE OF BREASTFEEDING

Sheila Kitzinger, LGSM, B.Litt., is a childbirth educator and social anthropologist. After training to teach drama and voice production, she read social anthropology at Oxford University, where she then carried out research on race relations, going on to teach and research at the University of Edinburgh.

Since 1958 she has been developing her Psychosexual Method and has studied preparation for childbirth and styles of childbearing in cultures as varied as those of the Caribbean, the United States, and Africa. In Britain she teaches couples and trains teachers for the National Childbirth Trust, of which she is on the Panel of Advisors, and is also a Consultant for the International Childbirth Education Association, and from 1971 to 1973 she held the Joost de Blank Award for research into the problems facing West Indian mothers in Britain. She has lectured widely in North America, South America, Israel, the Scandinavian countries, South Africa, and Australia. She is a Director of the Oxford Birth Centre.

Sheila Kitzinger's other books include *Giving Birth, The Parents' Emotions in Childbirth, Education and Counselling for Childbirth, The Place of Birth,* a study of the environment in which birth takes place (edited with Professor John Davis), *The Experience of Childbirth* (published by Penguin), *The Good Birth Guide,* a study of some three hundred maternity hospitals and women's experiences in them, *Women as Mothers,* a comparative anthropological study of mothers in different societies, and *Birth at Home.* She has also produced cassette tape recordings, *Journey Through Birth,* for couples working together to prepare themselves for childbirth.

She is married to Uwe Kitzinger, Dean of the European Institute of Business Administration at Fontainebleau. Their home is in Oxfordshire, England, and they have five daughters.

SHEILA KITZINGER

The Experience of
Breastfeeding

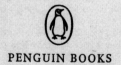

PENGUIN BOOKS

Penguin Books Ltd, Harmondsworth,
Middlesex, England
Penguin Books, 625 Madison Avenue,
New York, New York 10022, U.S.A.
Penguin Books Australia Ltd, Ringwood,
Victoria, Australia
Penguin Books Canada Limited, 2801 John Street,
Markham, Ontario, Canada L3R 1B4
Penguin Books (N.Z.) Ltd, 182–190 Wairau Road,
Auckland 10, New Zealand

First published in Great Britain
in Pelican Books 1979
First published in the United States of America
in Penguin Books 1980
Reprinted 1982

Printed in the United States of America by
Offset Paperback Mfrs., Inc., Dallas, Pennsylvania
Set in Intertype Lectura

Contents

Acknowledgements

I SHOULD like to thank Dr David Baum, Dr Aidan Macfarlane and Chloe Fisher, SRN, SCM, MTD, with whom I have had the opportunity to discuss many of the matters explored in these pages. Though I should stress that the opinions expressed are my own, they have always been stimulating in their views and helpful in their counsel.

Most of all I want to thank my family, especially my husband, Uwe, who gives constant loving support and encouragement, and our five daughters, all of whom have to bear with a mother suddenly hunting for a reference in the middle of a meal or retreating into her study because a deadline has to be met, or, it must be admitted, Jenny, has only half her mind on Elizabeth the First's foreign policy! I especially want to thank our daughters, too, for the way in which they have welcomed into the home new mothers who are encountering problems. They have always entertained the babies and kept them happy with such confidence and aplomb that I know that their own unselfconscious assurance has often given an anxious mother just the boost she needed.

To my secretary, Audrey Macefield, too, my most grateful thanks and admiration for her skills of fast and accurate typing and her flair for often knowing what I am about to say before I have said it!

A Note to the Reader

THE BABY: HE, SHE, IT?

I have never been able to decide what I ought to call the baby. In different books I have written I have called the baby 'he', 'he' and 'she' just about equally, and 'it'. As I have not yet called the baby 'she' and since I have myself had five daughters, I think it is about time the baby was called 'she' for the most part. I shall vary this occasionally as I do not want what I have to say about babies to seem irrelevant to boy babies. I apologize to the mothers of boys for this arbitrary piece of discrimination against the male.

YOUR PARTNER

I also use the term 'husband', partly because most mothers, either because they want them, or because they are subject to social pressures to have them, have babies with someone, who whether legally or not, is in fact a husband. I could have adopted the term 'consort', but that sounds a bit regal, or 'partner' which used throughout a book sounds too much like a western, or 'companion' which sounds plain dull! Although I realize that there are some mothers who face the challenge of parenthood on their own, I write on the whole for couples who are committed to each other, whether they think of themselves as husband and wife, or lovers, or friends who have a child together. I believe that it is very difficult to embark on the adventure of parenting without someone who loves you, and particularly hard on a new mother to face the tasks and emotional turmoil of child-rearing without someone who cherishes her when she needs it. For it is not enough for her to cherish her baby; if she is really to be able to give generously of her love *she* needs to be cherished too, and if she is emotionally undernourished this means that she has less to give to her baby. The dynamic, active relationship between the couple can be the rich store on which parenthood thrives and from which each can derive strength and fresh courage when everything is going wrong. This is just as true for a man and woman who are not bound by a legal certificate, or for two women who decide to have a child and bring it up together, as it is a husband and wife.

In some ways, too, the mother–child relationship is like a pressure cooker – intense, passionate and often explosive. When there is just one parent all the emotions are concentrated and passing between only two people. Although there may be difficulties in working out together and dovetailing parental roles, allowing these emotions to flow between two parents and more than one child permits a more relaxed atmosphere and lets each parent stand back, or even escape, occasionally, and thus get a better perspective on problems.

Commitment between the partners also means that each is in some way prepared for commitment to the child. For babies are non-returnable.

1. Learning about breastfeeding

It was a cocktail party and I had just refilled the charming Frenchman's glass. 'But,' he said, 'how can you possibly be writing a book about *breastfeeding*?' 'You mean, it should just come naturally?' 'Why, yes. My wife when she breastfed said that she felt like a *mammal*. She hated it, but she did it.'

I tried to explain that this book was about feelings as well as techniques, that it was also for women who found that it did not come quite as naturally as they had hoped, and for couples so that they could see breastfeeding in the context of their relationship together. 'Men? You write for men too?' he exclaimed. 'But how can it be anything to do with a man?'

It may seem odd to write a book about breastfeeding for a couple to read together. After all, interested as a man may be, he cannot himself breastfeed, and I concede that it is reasonable to ask if one is not stretching the notion of 'togetherness' too far in suggesting that he study the subject and do any more than register his general vague approval for the idea. But there is a strong case for a couple sharing this, as they shared the birth of the baby.

In my own experience I have found that over and over again a man's support for his wife during the time she is starting to feed their baby, his confidence in her and the basic knowledge he has of how lactation works, are decisive factors in her ability to breastfeed happily. This is why this book is for you both.

Breastfeeding *does* concern men. How they feel and talk about it affects a woman's attitude to what she is doing, her relationship with the baby and her sense of her own body as something which is loved and enjoyed by her husband or an object some aspects of which he finds distasteful. Breastfeeding is neither a question simply of producing enough milk nor one of somehow getting that milk into a baby. It is also a matter of the woman's emotions about using her breasts and her body for this purpose and of her partner's attitudes to her doing it too. These are central to whether or not she wants to and actually can breastfeed.

So although this book is about feeding a baby, it does not focus on the child so much as on the *relationship* between the mother and baby, the parents themselves and the father and baby. This different focus is important because so much that happens in child-rearing is itself an outcome of other processes that are occurring in the family and outside world. A baby is not brought up in a vacuum. It is born into a system of interaction already flowing between the parents, rather like a duet, which quickly changes to a trio in which the new-comer's notes are by far the most insistent. So I am writing not only about lactation, but also about the stresses and satisfactions of learning to live together in a new family.

There are other books about breastfeeding, why it is important and how to do it, but nothing specifically addressed to both the new parents as they sort out their life-style with a baby and their necessarily changed relationships with each other.

Birth is an intense and dramatic psychosexual experience, quite as much or even more so than love-making and inter-course. In the same way breastfeeding is psychosexual too, involving as it does a giving of the woman's body, release to let the milk flow, and relations between bodies, her own and the baby's. This is not to say that the feelings a woman has when giving the baby the breast are identical to or even similar to those she has when making love. They may be markedly different and are often quite distinct in her mind. Some women experience orgasms when breastfeeding. Probably most women do not. But orgasm is not the only pleasur-able experience in sexuality. We know that goal-oriented sex which looks to orgasmic release as the only 'successful' kind of climax tends to be self-defeating and often in the end strangely unsatisfying. Sex is much more than that and is composed of far more varied and subtle themes. The sense of the completeness of her own body, her satisfaction in giving, her closeness to and union with the baby as she breastfeeds, are some of these other aspects of sex, which are no less to be valued because they do not lead to orgasm.

Just as genital sex is not just what the man does to the woman or what she does to him, but of how they interact, so breastfeeding is the interaction between the mother and her baby. It is not therefore a question merely of techniques. You can use all the right techniques and yet find that things go wrong because there is something not right with the atmosphere or you are failing to respond to signals the baby is giving.

From the very start there is a pre-verbal 'language' with which the baby communicates with those caring for it if they look carefully enough. Psychologists have recently discovered a good deal about this relationship and the interaction that goes on, often at an unconscious level, between mother and baby, and for that matter between father and baby. Understanding something of what they have to say can help a mother become aware of her baby's needs so that she can adapt to her baby appropriately.

Since in early neonatal life babies need feeding very often, at least every four hours and sometimes almost continuously, a great part of this interaction concerns the feeding relationship that goes on during it and at intervals between sucking.

It is not only the interaction of mother and baby which is vital; the interaction of the couple also influences the feeding relationship positively or negatively and can often make all the difference between enjoying breastfeeding or hating it and between being able to or failing. This is not just a matter of the husband's superficial attitude, whether he approves and thinks his wife ought to try it or not, but of his deeper feelings about her role as a wife and as a mother and about her body in relation to the baby. The interaction of other members of the family, of people whose opinions you respect, those you encounter frequently from day to day and doctors, health visitors and midwives, can all be important too. And here too we can learn something from psychology and psychotherapy, so that we can know some at least of the irrational forces in human conduct which may influence breastfeeding and can have understanding, instead of resentment or irritation, when a husband seems almost jealous of the baby, a grandmother gives unsolicited advice about how to breastfeed, or when a professional adviser lays down the law about how you should breastfeed, having never done it herself.

There is one thing that a breastfeeding woman is never short of – advice. It pours in from all sides, from other women, from people who have breastfed successfully themselves and a great many others who have not, from the young and the old, from relatives and neighbours and casual contacts at the checkout in the supermarket or the queue in the post office. I hope that this book is not going to add to it! Ninety-nine per cent of it is superfluous and mothers get dithered and confused and sometimes bitterly distressed by it.

There probably is a place for advice, but not for the kind that tells a woman what she ought to do. *The advice that can be useful is the kind which describes a situation realistically, based on information the mother herself gives and observations she has made about her baby and her own reactions, mirrors this picture in as direct a way as possible and allows the mother to see the situation with a little more clarity. It helps us to sort out difficulties ourselves and is non-directive.* In my own experience very little advice given to the breastfeeding mother is of this kind.

There is certainly a place for a 'friendly ear'. Many difficulties can be solved if we avoid giving way to panic or becoming deluged with guilt about somehow failing the baby and failing as mothers, and instead talk through how we feel about what we are doing and sort out priorities. To do this you either have to be able to get behind a typewriter and write it all down or have somebody understanding and entirely non-judgemental to whom you can talk. This is where non-professional breastfeeding counsellors and friends come in. Their great skill is that they are prepared to listen and to give their time without thinking that it is wasted because they are not coming in and changing things *for* the mother who is facing difficulties with feeding.

It may seem trite to say that breastfeeding is natural. But

it is important to remember that the human race would not have survived unless it was and that all over the world, under very different climatic conditions, living in varied kinds of dwellings, eating vastly different kinds of food, resting or working hard in the fields, women have done it successfully. Many of these women have had no education as we know it and have certainly not understood how the mammary glands are constructed, and if we asked them how they did it they probably would not be able to give us one good idea! There is no secret 'trick of the trade'. The point is that lactation is a spontaneous physiological process and breastfeeding a natural act. And yet it is undeniable that many women in modern urban post-industrial society face problem after problem when breastfeeding. There is an analogy with sex here too, of course. Orgasm is a spontaneous physiological process and comes quite naturally without people having to take lessons in it or learn special techniques. Yet many men and women in Western society face difficulties with it and have to go back and find out how to clear away the barriers. The research and sexual therapy developed by William Masters and Virginia Johnson[1] has shown that this can be done and that people can rediscover joy in their bodies and learn how to live fully through them. I believe that we can do much the same with breastfeeding, using techniques not as ends in themselves, but as stations on the way to being able to fully *give* ourselves in breastfeeding.

2. Is human milk good enough for babies?

Each mammal produces the kind of milk best suited to the needs of its young. Aquatic mammals, such as whales, seals and porpoises produce high-energy milks – important because their babies tend to lose heat rapidly in the water. The blue whale, for example, makes milk which is 50 per cent fat, compared with human milk which is only approximately 4·5 per cent fat. High-energy milks are also produced by some small land mammals, such as rabbits and tree shrews, who suckle infrequently. A tree shrew mother feeds her baby for only five minutes in every two days.[1]

Low-solute milk is typical of mammals who suckle their babies almost continuously. Human milk has one of the lowest solute and protein concentrations.[2] All primates produce milk much lower in protein than it might be thought they needed on the basis of body size. This reflects their relatively slow growth rates. Human milk is approximately 1 per cent protein, whereas rabbit's milk has a protein content of 10–13 per cent. It takes a rat or rabbit only about six days to double its birth weight, a piglet about ten days and a puppy about eleven days. A calf grows at a slower rate than this and takes ten to eleven weeks to double its size. But a chimpanzee takes a little over fourteen weeks, and a breast-fed human baby about twenty-seven weeks, though there are wide variations. (A baby fed on artificial milk tends to double its birthweight much more rapidly and may do so in about fifteen weeks.)

Cow's milk is very different from human milk in other ways too. The contrast is so great that it has even been suggested that it would be better to base artificial milk for babies on that from another mammal whose milk is more like human milk. Otters have been suggested! Precise comparisons are difficult because neither cow's nor human milk are standardized products. Breast milk varies between women, at different stages from the onset of lactation until its conclusion, with different babies (strong suckers producing a different kind of milk from those who only suck weakly, for example), between different feeds within the twenty-four hours and at the beginning and end of each feed. It is important to bear in mind that all the comparative figures given in the following pages are approximate, and that it is impossible to discover what human milk is simply by making a list of the properties of a series of samples. Since it changes at different times and according to the baby's needs, it must really be studied in terms of the biological *interaction* between the mother's breast and the baby.

All milk is beautifully adapted to the needs of the growing young of the species. Human milk as it is at present in the evolutionary cycle has evolved to suit creatures whose main characteristic is the development of a relatively large brain with special growth of the frontal lobes. This is why the protein content of human milk is much lower than cow's milk and why nutrients which assist brain development are present in significant quantities. Breast milk is designed not for creatures who are strong as oxen, as large as elephants, or who grow as fast as rabbits, but for beings whose cortical development permits them to explore, invent, form families, evolve new kinds of social organization and cultures and through speech, reading and writing, share with others and hand on through history their values, experiences and discoveries, and who have a potential for abstract thought and the concepts embodied in mathematics, science, religion and philosophy.

Human milk is biochemically unique. More than a hundred constituents have now been isolated and still more are being discovered every year. In 1966 alone six new polysaccharides were found to exist in breast milk.[3]

Human milk is adjusted to a particular baby's needs at that phase of its growth. I have mentioned already that it varies from day to day, between morning and evening and from feed to feed. The milk produced at the onset of lactation also has a very different fat/protein/carbohydrate ratio from that produced after the mother has been lactating for several months, and it continues to change as she carries on breast-feeding.

The process starts with the formation of *colostrum*. This is the kind of milk present in the breasts before delivery. It is a yellowish liquid which looks like cream on the top of rich milk, and is very high in *protein*. It also contains *antibodies* against a wide range of diseases, including polio, influenza, the Coxsacki group of viruses and salmonella. The newborn baby's gut is immunologically very vulnerable and colostrum has an extremely important function in providing a kind of primer of protective paint[4] with this immunoglobu-lin-rich fluid which contains both 1gG and 1gA in concentrations much higher than those of the mother's blood. Without such protection the baby is exposed to bacterial, viral gut and respiratory infections. Also, large molecules of protein can reach the intestinal tissues and produce an immune response in the bottle-fed baby whose gut lining has not been 'primed' by colostrum, thus causing cow's milk allergy, which we shall discuss later. Colostrum has a laxative effect and helps to clear out the meconium (the first bowel movements) already in the baby's intestines at birth.

Cows have their own type of colostrum, but this is not used for babies artificially fed from birth. It is usually given to calves because it is important in cattle rearing. When newborn calves are removed from their mothers and fed by other cows they suffer a high mortality from gastroenteritis. Even if cow's colostrum were available for newborn babies, the infections met by a cow would be unlikely to produce antibodies against human illnesses. Pasteurization destroys the immunoglobins both in colostrum and in mature milk.

Colostrum is gradually replaced by *transitional milk* over a period of several days, starting on the third to fifth day after the birth. The mother may get anxious that she is losing the quality of her milk, because the originally creamy fluid is streaked with a thinner, more watery-looking liquid. This transitional milk is also high in *protein* and contains many *immunoglobins*.

By the end of about a week (that is, ten days to two weeks after the birth) this has changed to *mature milk*, which has a lower protein content. It usually has a bluish colour, like watered-down cow's milk, and it is at this stage that a woman who is not given encouragement and emotional support may have serious doubts about whether her milk is 'rich' or 'strong' enough, especially when she sees the drops of milk leaking at the beginning of a feed. Yet a mother's milk cannot be too weak for her baby. This is exactly how it should look.

This watery milk gives way to whiter, high calory milk towards the *end* of each feed. The fat content may increase from as low as just over 1 per cent at the onset to over 8 per cent at the end, and the protein content by one and a half times. So mature milk varies in appearance according to whether it is the beginning or end of a feed. But during the feed, the *rate of flow* is reduced. This means that during any single feed most of the protein and sugar are taken by the baby when the flow is fast in the first five minutes or so. A continuous analysis of one mother–baby pair revealed that the baby took 60 per cent of the total milk volume and the protein in the first five minutes of one feed, 40 per cent of the fat and more than 50 per cent of the total energy. In the following six minutes the baby received 26 per cent of the volume, 25 per cent of the protein, carbohydrate and total energy, and 33 per cent of the fat. In the next seven minutes the baby had 13 per cent of the volume, 10 per cent of the protein and energy and 25 per cent of the fat.[5]

In the first few days of life, following on an initial wide-awake period immediately following delivery, the baby may sleep nearly all the time. After that she tends to have more frequent and longer waking times. This does not mean that the milk is inadequate. The baby is interacting with her environment and needs to be awake in order to learn. Unfortunately this usually coincides with the production of the watery-looking mature milk and the combination of a crying baby and this bluish milk leads the mother to think that she is failing at breastfeeding.

During the first week it is normal for the baby who is

being fed naturally to lose weight. The birth weight is not usually regained until the baby is ten days to two weeks old. A weight loss at this time does not mean that anything is wrong, provided that weight starts to be put on at about ten days.

Right through the process of lactation changes occur in breast milk as it adapts itself to the baby's needs. As the baby grows the milk becomes more thirst-quenching, contains less protein and is available in larger quantities for the vigorously sucking baby. As she goes on growing the fat content of the milk becomes less, so that after five to six months of lactation it is reduced to only about 2 per cent.[6] The production of breast milk is dynamic.

I have mentioned already that the rate at which milk flows also varies. At the beginning of a feed it is fast; towards the end it is slow. The baby has to work harder for what it wants. The constantly changing nature and rate of flow in human milk may be related to an appetite-control mechanism which helps a baby to feel full up and satisfied as the milk increases in fat content and the flow slows down and teaches her when to stop. It is a kind of 'anti-obesity system'.[7] A breastfed baby does not stop only when the breast is empty. The mother of a bottle-fed baby tends to jiggle him, shake the bottle and try to persuade him to finish because the formula has been made up in the estimated correct quantity for a baby of this age. Perhaps this, as well as the actual composition of cow's milk, explains why bottle-fed babies are more likely to be fat and their bodies to build extra fat cells which remain with them as adults to cause a weight problem.

The change in the rate of breast-milk flow also has the effect of allowing time for gastric emptying, and thus reducing the chances of colic. The bottle-fed baby receives all its milk at the same rate, which depends on the size of the hole in the teat.

The types of protein and the other food values in human milk are also different from those in cow's milk. It is not just a question of the proportions but of the kinds of protein, fat and sugar. Rolles draws the analogy between trying to imitate human milk and trying to design artificial blood: 'One might take a list of the chemical composition of homogenized human blood and make this synthetically by simply adding together the relevant constituents and claiming that you would have a blood substitute.'[8]

FATS

Both kinds of milk have about the same amount of fat, but the composition of fatty acids is radically different and a breastfed baby has a different 'fat profile' in its blood from that of a bottle-fed baby. Cow's milk contains a high proportion of saturated fatty acids. Human milk has high levels of unsaturated or short-chain fatty acids, especially linoleic acid, of which there may be eight times as much. When making artificial baby milk, the only way of changing the fats in cow's milk to short-chain fats is to introduce vegetable oils. So the baby food firms usually take the milk which is left over after cheese-making and add vegetable oil and vitamins and minerals to it. (If they no longer had markets in baby food they would have to find something else to do with these by-products.)

Ninety-two per cent of the fat in breast milk is absorbed by the baby. This is because the smaller a fatty acid the higher the solubility of its salts. In human milk the large-molecular-weight fatty acids tend to be in the middle of the molecule, the smaller ones being on the outside.[9] Breast milk is rich in *lipase*, which liberates free fatty acids from the triglycerides and produces energy. The baby cannot absorb the fats in cow's milk so easily and failure to digest them also reduces the absorption of calcium.

Autopsies on young Americans killed in Korea revealed the startling fact that a large percentage of them displayed the early signs of coronary artery disease. These young men came from a culture in which the vast majority of babies were artificially fed. Adults with heart disease have been shown to have high levels of antibodies to cow's milk. It looks as if an immunological reaction to cow's milk may occur early on and continue throughout life, causing disturbance in fatty acid metabolism, making the platelets sticky and laying the foundations for coronary heart disease.

The *cholesterol* level in breast milk is also much higher than in cow's milk. This may help the myelinization of the central nervous system and the development of enzyme systems in the baby.[10] In spite of the bad press that cholesterol has had, this is one time in life when cholesterol is good for you! It may be that cholesterol in breast milk enables human beings to handle cholesterol better later on.

PROTEIN

We have seen that cow's milk is much richer in protein than is human milk. It contains at least three times as much protein as breast milk because calves need to grow at a much greater rate than human babies. New, more precise ways of measuring protein suggest that human milk may contain even less than previously thought, approximately 0·88 per cent.[11] We have seen also that the *kind* of protein is different. Cow's milk protein has a high rate of casein in relation to lactalbumin (4·5:1). The casein–lactalbumin ratio in human milk is about 1:2. The casein produces a *curd*. That of cow's milk is far greater in quantity than the curd produced by human milk, a distinction which can easily be noted by a mother on examining the baby's stools if she has switched to an artificial milk feed. Whereas the curd of human milk is soft, that from cow's milk is firm and of a rubbery consistency. The stools produced by the two milks also have characteristically different odours. Breast-milk stools smell sweet and are unobjectionable. The stools of a baby fed on cow's milk tend to be grey, lumpy and foul smelling. It is this harder curd, especially if a baby has been given over-concentrated feeds, with an extra scoop added to 'enrich' the feed, that readily leads to constipation and pain on passing stools in an artificially fed baby. A breastfed baby, even though it may have bowel motions only once every few days or longer, does not get constipated, and the stools remain mustard-like until solid foods or supplementary milks are introduced. The breastfed baby's stools are *acid*, and an acid medium is unfavourable for the growth of bacteria which cause gastro-enteritis. Bottle-fed babies have alkaline stools. This is a favourable environment for the growth of pathogenic organisms.

There are other differences between the different kinds of protein too which make cow's milk harder for a baby to digest. 'Humanizing' cow's milk does not produce an accurate copy of breast milk even so far as the protein content is concerned.

Breast milk contains carrier proteins, one of which, *lactoferrin*, is bound with iron. This permits all the iron available in human milk to be absorbed by the baby and yet, because it is tightly linked with the protein, does not let it break loose and nourish pathogenic bacteria. Baby-food manufacturers have not been able to mimic lactoferrin, and instead just add large quantities of iron to the formula. It is possible that lactoferrin is bound to other minerals too, so facilitating their complete absorption by the baby, but a good deal of research still remains to be done on this.

All protein is composed of *amino acids*. The amino acid content of breast and cow's milk is very different. Breast milk contains a high proportion of *cystine*, and another amino acid, *taurine*, which is not present in cow's milk at all and which studies of rats demonstrate is taken up by the brain in the first few days after birth.

We do not yet know all the properties of breast milk, and when a new constituent is discovered often do not understand why it should be there. This is particularly the case with the amino acids, the different forms of casein and the nucleotides and glycoproteins.[12]

SUGAR

Sugar in the milk of all mammals is in the form of *lactose*. There is nearly twice as much lactose in human milk as there is in cow's milk. This is why when cow's milk was first modified by infant-food manufacturers extra sugar was added. Unfortunately this was often sucrose, a much sweeter form of sugar, which trains the baby's palate to expect sweet food. When sucrose is metabolized it may disturb sugar-regulating mechanisms and precipitate diabetes in later life. It also encourages the growth of abnormal bacteria in the gut.[13] If another sugar, fructose, is introduced instead, the baby cannot readily metabolize it.

Lactose assists in the development of the central nervous system, increases calcium absorption and bone growth, creates relatively acid stools and nourishes intestinal lactobaccilli which fight the micro-organisms of disease and which play a role in the digestion of carbohydrates.

VITAMINS

The vitamin content of breast milk depends on the vitamin content of the mother's diet. *Vitamins A, C and K* are those which the poorly nourished mother is most likely to lack and which may need supplementing during pregnancy and lactation. Breast milk has more *vitamin A and C* than cow's milk, and breastfed babies do not need extra vitamins until they are at least six months old. Human milk also has *vitamin E*, which is not present in cow's milk, and *vitamin B_{12}*, which, though in cow's milk, takes a different form. It used to be thought that there was very little *vitamin D* in human milk, but water-soluble vitamin D has now been discovered to be present, which brings the total content up to that found in vitamin-D-fortified cow's milk.[14]

MINERALS

Cow's milk has many more minerals than breast milk, about six times as much phosphorus, nearly four times as much calcium and almost four times as much sodium (salt). It produces a great solute load for the baby's renal system so that blood urea levels are far higher than those of a breastfed baby. What is happening is that they are accumulating as waste products in the baby's tissues.[15] If softened water is used to make up artificial foods the sodium may be increased by as much as 50 per cent.[16]

The result is that breastfed babies are *biochemically different* from artificially fed babies. The bottle-fed baby is more likely to retain fluids, gain weight and look plump because the tissues are swollen with sodium and water. This does not matter very much unless the baby has diarrhoea and becomes dehydrated as a result, when blood urea, serium sodium and potassium levels can become dangerously high and cause kidney damage. Sodium poisoning harms the growing brain and can even kill.

The baby receiving large amounts of salt usually gets very thirsty and cries. The mother then gives more of the artificial milk and since she may interpret the crying as being one of hunger, is tempted to make up the feed with more powder than before, thus giving the baby still more salt. It is a vicious circle.

Breast milk contains far less *calcium* than cow's milk. The high proportion of calcium in unmodified cow's milk, the absorption of which is further assisted by the large amounts of phosphorus, can produce convulsions (hypocalcaemic tetany). This is another reason why it is dangerous to put in extra scoops of dried milk and why the thing the bottle-fed baby most lacks may be plain water. Although human milk contains less calcium, that which is present is absorbed completely. This is because the kind of fat in the milk determines the absorbability of calcium in the gut. When acids are low in molecular weight, as they are in breast milk, the calcium soaps formed by the action of lipase on fat are soluble. In cow's milk, however, much of the calcium usually passes out in the faeces, which is fortunate in view of its danger for the baby.

IRON

A full-term baby is born with about 75 mg of iron – which has been stored in the liver prenatally – for each kilogram of body weight. This is sufficient for use until the birth weight has been doubled, usually between four and six months of age. (A premature baby often doubles the birth weight by the time it is eight to ten weeks old.) From that time on the growing baby needs iron in whatever food is given. It is no good giving this in a form in which it cannot be absorbed by the baby's intestinal tract, as is the case with Popeye's famous spinach.

Milk does not contain much iron, only about 0·5 to 1·0 mg a quart, and there is little difference between the iron content of breast and cow's milk. But there is a remarkable difference in the way the baby *absorbs* the iron. As long ago as 1928[17] it was discovered that breastfed babies had a higher haemoglobin level than bottle-fed babies. As we have seen already, breast milk contains a protein, lactoferrin, which binds iron tightly.

Paediatricians working in New York studied babies who had received breast milk only for the first six to eighteen months of life, and whose mothers received no supplementary iron. None of them was anaemic.[18] They then studied the absorption of radioactive iron in breast and cow's milk using adult volunteers. Two weeks after the subjects had drunk one kind of milk or another their blood was tested, and it was discovered that at least 20 per cent of the iron taken with human milk had been absorbed, but only 13 per cent of the iron in cow's milk. Since adults absorb only about half as much iron as babies, a breastfed baby is going to absorb still more. Further studies in Finland fixed this figure at nearly 50 per cent of the iron in breast milk compared with 10 per cent of that in unfortified cow's milk and approximately 4 per cent of the iron in fortified formula.[19] A baby needs to absorb altogether 140mg of iron in its first year. The breastfed baby uses about 0·4mg of iron for every quart of milk and this comes to about 146mg for the first year of life. A bottle-fed baby gets nothing like this amount, not because it is not present in the milk, but because it is not absorbed.

Very high protein feeds reduce absorption of iron. The presence of lactose and vitamin C in breast milk also assists absorption. Phosphorus, however, of which there is more in cow's milk, inhibits absorption. When babies are given other foods as well as milk they may have reduced iron absorption both because of the combination of foods and also because they tend to take less milk once they are given solids. It looks as if this is not a good thing, at least from the point of view of the iron the baby is getting, and we can conclude that a fully breastfed baby does not need extra iron.

If iron supplements are added to human milk it loses a large part of its property of protecting the baby against diarrhoea, because some pathogenic micro-organisms in the intestines live on iron. This is especially serious in hot countries, where standards of hygiene are low, or where there are epidemics of infantile diarrhoea.

When there is infection the haemoglobin level of the body normally drops. This has usually been considered a bad thing and doctors have often prescribed supplementary iron to raise the haemoglobin level. But research in Africa suggests that the drop in haemoglobin level may be a normal adaptive response of the human body, in a way similar to that in which a drop in temperature is adaptive in shock.

So it is neither necessary nor desirable to give a breastfed baby iron supplements until it is at least four or five months old.

FLUORIDE

The level of fluoride in breast milk varies with the amount in the mother's drinking water. Cow's milk contains much more and the artificially fed baby may receive fifty times as much as the breastfed baby. La Leche advises against the breastfeeding mother taking additional fluoride, however, since some babies have allergic reactions to it.

COPPER AND ZINC

Breast milk contains valuable trace elements which are present, but in lower amounts, in cow's milk. There is, for example, more copper in human than in cow's milk. One American study indicated that the ratio of zinc to copper may be important in relation to coronary heart disease in adults.[20] The zinc/copper ratio in human milk is much lower than that in cow's milk and as we have seen already, breastfed babies are less likely to suffer heart disease when they grow up.

Zinc reserves, unlike iron, are low in the newborn baby,

who thus depends on getting zinc in the diet. Although cow's milk contains zinc, it is bound to a large protein, whereas in human milk it is bound to a small protein and so is more readily available to the baby.[21] Babies fed on artificial milk containing less than 2mg per litre of zinc may fail to thrive. Sometimes a baby becomes really ill. There is an inherited disorder, acrodermatitis enteropathica, which results in skin lesions, diarrhoea and hair dropping out, associated with lack of zinc in the baby's diet.[22] The newborn baby cannot easily transport zinc in its intestines and so depends on a high concentration of zinc-binding protein in its milk. There is an especially high concentration of zinc in human colostrum.

ALLERGIES

We have already seen that another problem with cow's milk is that some babies and older children are allergic to it. No one knows the extent of cow's milk allergy, but a few babies actually die from it. This is why babies are sometimes fed on goat milk or a soy 'milk' instead of ordinary formula. It is not generally realized, however, that allergy to soya beans is not uncommon.

Cow's milk allergy may be a much underdiagnosed condition because it often presents in ways other than milk intolerance. One study. done with children aged between eleven months and seventeen years who were allergic to cow's milk, revealed that they had problems such as constipation, vomiting, colic, growth retardation and eczema; over 90 per cent of milk-allergic children suffer from rhinitis and asthma.[23] In a series of seventy-nine children who were milk allergic twenty-seven had psychological disturbances too. All these symptoms disappeared when cow's milk was omitted from their diet. Babies born to parents one or both of whom suffer from allergies are more likely to have an allergy to cow's milk than those of parents who have no allergies. This suggests that parents who themselves have allergies would be wise to avoid cow's milk completely and breastfeed until the child is able to drink from a cup, and that even then the effect of cow's milk should be carefully noted and should be introduced experimentally at first.

Indications that a bottle-fed baby, or one who is being 'topped up' with bottles, may have an allergy to cow's milk are feeding difficulties, either hard stools or loose, violent bowel actions, and vomiting, which may be projectile and is sometimes incorrectly diagnosed as being due to pyloric stenosis. These babies do not thrive and often have stuffy noses with a chronic loose-sounding cough[24] which is not cleared up by antibiotics. Eczema appears within the first three months, affecting first the inside of the elbows and legs and the wrists and behind the ears, soon extending to the neck, face and trunk. As the child gets older this becomes scaly and the child may also have recurrent tummy-aches and constipation. To test whether this is indeed a cow's milk allergy all forms of milk, including yoghurt, cheese and butter, should be omitted from the child's diet for an experimental period. If the symptoms abate milk and milk products should then be reintroduced to see if this will clinch the case. (Skin tests are unreliable.)

'HUMANIZED' MILK

Most babies can handle cow's milk well provided it is suitably modified by adding extra sugar, boiling, drying or evaporating it so that the protein is more easily digested and diluting it with water. But premature and low-birth-weight babies, and even a healthy full-term baby in the first six weeks of life, may have digestive upsets and, if the feeds are incorrectly made up, can even become seriously ill.

The most dangerous thing to do with baby formula, apart from the ever-present risk of infection with bottle feeding if hygiene is poor, is, as we have already seen, to reconstitute the milk in too concentrated a form so that the baby gets an excessive amount of minerals and becomes hypernatraemic because of the high mineral load. If this is done over a prolonged period brain cells are deprived of fluid and there is brain damage.

All proprietary milks have a high mineral content, fats and proteins which are not ideally suited to a baby's digestive system and inadequate vitamins unless they are 'humanized'. But as we have seen, 'humanizing' milk does not turn it into human milk. No one has yet succeeded in doing this. What humanizing does is to break down cow's milk into its constituents and combine them in a different way, still with a rather higher mineral content, with a proportion or all of the butterfat replaced with vegetable oil, sometimes with the protein changed to a mixture of skimmed cow's milk and electrodialysed whey (a process similar to that used in kidney machines) and the sugar changed to lactose or maltodextrin.[25] Other things, like iron and vitamins A, D and C are added either because breast milk contains more of these or because they are present in a more readily assimilatable form. The Oppé Report, *Present Day Practices in Infant Feeding*, raised the question, however, of whether in doing this, other important constituents of breast milk which have not yet been discovered may be destroyed.[26] At our present stage of knowledge, human milk cannot be duplicated. Moreover, even if we were able to mimic it by altering and adding to the constituents of cow's milk, we should still not have an exact substitute because of the way in which human milk adapts itself to the individual baby's needs.

AN ACTIVE IMMUNOLOGICAL ORGAN

I have heard human milk described as 'a transfer mechanism between total dependence and immunological independence'.[27] Fresh breast milk is not just a mixture of solid and liquid inanimate substances. It is a living fluid, abundant in microscopic organisms (enzymes, hormones and active cells) which promote health. These not only ensure the normal colonization of the gastro-intestinal tract but also fight invading pathogenic micro-organisms. So it is very important for the baby's defence against infection.[28]

When human milk is injected into mice given lethal doses of *Staphylococcus aureus* they are able to fight the infection.[29] When there are outbreaks of gastro-enteritis in maternity hospitals, breastfed infants are both less likely to suffer from the disease and, if they do get it, are less likely to die as a result.[30]

The cow is also able to protect its calf against infection (but not, of course, when its milk is fed to the young of other species). Research on cow's milk demonstrates that this is not simply a *passive* immunity, through antibodies in the milk which are resistant to disease to which the mother animal herself is immune, but that the mammary gland of the mother cow is itself an *immunological organ*.[31] The human breast is also able to react to microbes brought to it by the baby and to manufacture antibodies to fight infection. This is one reason why breastfed babies have fewer respiratory and gastro-intestinal infections than those fed on artificial milk.

A study done in a small town in New York State followed the progress of all healthy, full-term babies born in one month in one particular hospital for a period of a year, where good paediatric and other medical services were available to all the families.[32] This research showed that artificially fed babies had twice as many ear infections as breastfed babies, sixteen times more chest colds and two and a half times more gastro-intestinal upsets. The bottle-fed babies were admitted to hospital eight and a half times as often as breastfed babies. Overall, there was three and a half times more illness in bottle-fed than in breastfed babies.

Older babies who were breastfed longer than four and a half months became ill half as often as those breastfed less than four and a half months and those who were completely bottle-fed, independent of the educational level of the parents. This is particularly interesting because although it is widely recognized that it is much safer for poor families to breastfeed, it is often claimed that mothers who have education and live under good conditions do not expose their babies to any increased risk of illness if they choose to bottle-feed. If the results of this study are borne out by further research in other places this assumption is completely false.

All the evidence suggests that human milk is best to protect the baby in its journey from the growth period inside the uterus through the period of growth outside the uterus during which it develops to the point where it can function as a separate organism. Your breast milk is not only good enough for your baby; it is the perfect food throughout the first year of life.

3. The case for bottle feeding

There is one powerful argument for bottle feeding: that the mother herself prefers to do it that way. No other reasons for bottle feeding approach anywhere near the strength of such a statement and if a mother wishes to bottle feed it is her right to do so. She should be able to do this without being made to feel guilty. The choice is hers. Her breasts belong to her.

Yet often the expectant mother or the one who has just had a baby begins to feel that perhaps her body does not really belong to her. It belongs to doctors and nurses, to the hospital where the baby is born, to people who know better what is good for babies than she can herself, to the crowd of experts in something or other who seem to loom over her body as she progresses through pregnancy and labour and faces up to the challenge of being an adequate mother to this new and rather frightening baby. In pregnancy her body is poked and prodded and explored, tested and assessed: then in labour it is 'managed' by the obstetrician, perhaps wired up to electronic machines, linked by tubes to drips, injected by substances which make her drowsy and out of control. After delivery she is stitched, lying while a masked and gowned figure at the other end does careful embroidery around her vagina. No wonder she feels as if she needs to have her body back again and that she wants it to be *hers*. It is understandable that it can seem just too much to be required also to give her breasts to this incredibly savage little stranger who opens its mouth to grip her nipple between its jaws.

Somebody says, 'But *surely* you want to give your baby the best you can? ...' 'Poor little love; his mother doesn't want to breastfeed ...' Or if the mother produces excuses like 'I really think I haven't got enough milk' or 'The baby never seems satisfied' a kindly person may make all sorts of helpful suggestions which entirely miss the point that in her heart of hearts she does not *want* to breastfeed.

It is doubtful whether feeling she *ought* to have an orgasm ever actually helped a woman to get one. Similarly, feeling that one *ought* to breastfeed does not actually make it any easier.

In British hospitals today there is a great upsurge of interest in breastfeeding and many staff on postnatal wards are enthusiastic and approach the subject with an almost missionary zeal. This is splendid for those women who have already decided that they want to breastfeed and who are highly motivated. It creates difficulties for those women who for one reason or another are holding back from the experience and are seeking to protect themselves from it. We do not have to look any deeper than the hospital environment in which the vast majority of women nowadays have to bear their babies and to what is done to them there to understand how a woman may have an overwhelming need to *reclaim* her body.

It is important that antenatally it should be made quite clear to each woman that *she* can decide how to feed her baby, and that there are realistic alternatives. On the other hand, it is not enough to ask a woman, 'Breast or bottle?' and leave it at that. She may not have a clue as to what she wants. In a society where girls growing up gain very little experience of small babies and often even less experience of breastfeeding, expectant mothers need to learn about possible options, and some of the difficulties that may be encountered with each method of feeding. Nor should it be a question of someone in a white coat standing up in front of a class and giving information. Expectant mothers, and fathers too, will probably want to talk with others and discuss not only facts but feelings too. These feelings should include those which may assail the new parents after the birth, both in the immediate postpartum days and in the early weeks. A baby inside the uterus is still a neat little package; the newborn baby can easily seem a hostile stranger and a bundle of energy which is completely out of the parents' control.

In antenatal classes I sometimes discuss with parents the ways in which they think about the baby who is still inside and the fantasies they may have about it: the sex, whether it is dark or fair, fat or thin, contented or discontented, energetic or rather passive, cuddly or not. Even the joke name that many expectant parents give the foetus suggests the way they perceive the unborn baby. Sometimes we go on from there to use our imaginations and to project ourselves into the future, after the baby is born: 'Imagine yourself after the baby has come, perhaps about three weeks old. Think of a good scene, like a short scene from a play, in which everything is just as you want it to be. How would you describe it?' After we have discussed this I suggest that we turn our thoughts to a very different scene and think of everything going badly. Anticipatory fantasies like these allow expectant parents to think ahead, and perhaps what is even more important, *feel* ahead. They can be the means by which the couple can make some emotional preparation for the enormous changes which will occur with the birth of the baby. It is interesting, however, that a couple who have not yet had their baby (and who have not had one before) still see themselves as the main actors on the scene in these anticipatory dramas. The baby is an object, of care and attention, love and concern, but still very much something which is acted on, rather than a living being who herself is one of the chief protagonists in a triangle of supercharged emotions.

It is this which comes as such a shock to many new mothers. The reality and vitality of one's baby can be very exciting, but it is also challenging and can be alarming. In my experience some of the difficulties which a woman encounters initially in breastfeeding relate to this sense of dynamic otherness of the baby, and she needs to talk about it. This is one of the things a breastfeeding counsellor should enable her to do. It often helps too if a couple discuss it together. The feelings she has may be too powerful for her to handle while at the same time making attempts to breastfeed. She only feels 'safe' when she can give the baby a bottle. She is protected then not only from the baby's demands on her, but also from the feeling that she cannot give enough, cannot be an adequate mother and that to try to do so is like 'getting blood out of a stone', a metaphor which is extraordinarily appropriate to the woman who is straining to breastfeed but who feels she cannot, if only because her holding back from the baby means that the nipple is not inserted deep enough into the baby's mouth, becomes sore and cracked and may start to bleed.

What I am really saying here is that it is not enough to encourage women to breastfeed and to give advice, nor even to give loving support. We also have to accept the reality and validity of each woman's own feelings about the relation between her body and the baby, and that these are just as much facts as are the shape of the nipples and the baby's weight gain. A woman who says she wants to breastfeed but is basically uncomfortable about it should be able to feel that she is free to do what she really wants, based on her own experience at the time, and that she will be given support for whatever she decides.

The odd thing is that when emotional support of this kind is given a woman is much more likely to try breastfeeding and to continue because she likes it, than if she is in an atmosphere where she feels she *ought* to breastfeed. I have sometimes said to an expectant mother who has expressed doubts about breastfeeding (or one who has said to me, for example, 'I'm not sure that I'll be able to do it because I don't like my breasts being touched anyway', or 'It may seem silly, but I feel that my breasts are for my husband. I don't think I'd ever feel the same about them if I let the baby suck them') 'It sounds to me as if bottle feeding might be the right choice for you.' Yet I have never yet had one woman to whom I have spoken like this who did not decide to breastfeed, and end up enjoying it.

There are other women to whom I have not spoken in this way, because I had not picked up clues about their feelings and only discovered them later, who have encountered insuperable difficulties with breastfeeding. I wish now that I had spoken in this way to more of them. For in a society in which pregnancy and birth are taken over by large in-

stitutions and modern technology, one in which the woman
is increasingly alienated from her own body as it passes
through the myriad changes involved in the process of childbearing, women need to be 'given permission' to use their
breasts as they wish and a genuine choice of breast or bottle
feeding.

SOME OTHER REASONS FOR PREFERRING BOTTLE FEEDING

*'It is all very well to talk about doing things naturally. But
we do not live in a natural world. If we did we should not
give penicillin to a baby with pneumonia, but just let it die.
The "natural" argument about breastfeeding does not hold
water.'*

This is usually a man talking, but some women, especially
those who are concerned to liberate themselves from
'woman's biological destiny' may explain a reluctance to
breastfeed in the same way. It is a valid argument. The point
is that we each have to decide what aspects of 'the natural'
we value in our personal lives. There are usually times when
all of us feel a great sense of relief and refreshment at being
able to get back to natural things, whether these are the
countryside or the sea, smelling grass, hay, leaves and
flowers, or the salt spray, hearing the rustling of insects,
the wind and birds' cries, seeing sky and water and the shape
of the land. And we often feel the sense of glad return when
we do things that are spontaneous rather than contrived and
carefully worked out, and get back to engaging in activities
which involve our bodies and hands rather than working with
machinery or being bound at a desk. Most of all there can
be deep satisfaction in being in an intimate and rewarding
relationship with another human being, rather than just with
things.

This is what breastfeeding is all about. It is 'natural' in
this sense. It is not the only way of relating to a baby but
it is one which can feel as if the surge of life which manifests
itself in all natural creation, and in human love, is flowing

through you too. Some women never get this feeling; but for others it is a vivid reality. It may be possible to experience the same thing when giving a baby a bottle.

'*I didn't manage to do it last time and I want to avoid all the fuss and bother that there was then.*'

Again, this is a valid reason for not engaging in a long struggle. But there is probably a case for seeing what happens next time. It may be very different. Simply having a more relaxed attitude may help. The mother also probably learned from the last experience and realizes some of the mistakes that were made then. She can make a note of them before the baby is born so that they are clear in her mind, and can also explain to anybody who is helping her just why she wants to do things differently this time.

'*I have inverted nipples and have been told that the baby won't be able to get them into its mouth properly.*'

Babies cope with the most surprisingly flat, lopsided or retracted nipples. If the mother can get the nipple to stand out a bit by touching it or asking her husband to caress it the baby will do the rest of the work by drawing it out further When the mother longs to feed because the baby is crying or she can feel his cheek against the breast she will find, too, that the nipple will become erect by itself, just as the clitoris becomes erect when she is sexually excited. There is more about inverted nipples on page 44.

You do not have to have nipples like bottle teats to be able to breastfeed. Small nipples do very well. They will get larger during the time a mother is feeding and afterwards will go back to their previous size.

'*I am very flat-chested, and always have been, so there is not much chance that I shall be able to breastfeed. Perhaps it is not worth trying.*'

The size of the breasts has nothing to do with the amount of glandular tissue in them, which is the only part of the breast which is relevant to milk production. The rest is all fat and connective tissue, however large the breasts. In some ways a small breast is easier to handle and to lift into the baby's mouth neatly. In early pregnancy breasts undergo changes to prepare them for breastfeeding and tend to get larger. If a woman notices this happening it is a good sign that she will be able to breastfeed if she wants to.

'My husband isn't at all keen on the idea. He thinks it mucky.'

Only the woman herself knows the relationship she has with her husband and how her decision about this can affect it. Certainly she has to take it into the reckoning. It may be worth asking him if he thinks he could handle his feelings about it for a couple of months or so, when it is a great advantage to a baby's health to be breastfed. It is important to discuss this with him because the couple need to work it out together, and if they fail to do so the woman will not only feel that she does not have his support, but that feeding the baby is almost an act of aggression against him. He will probably want to learn some facts about breastfeeding and can find these in Chapter 2. Some men cannot face the night-time feed, especially if it takes place in *their* bed. If so, the mother might organize herself so that she can lie on a couch or divan in another room for night feeds, and have a system where the feed given just before they go to bed takes place while he is in the bath or working in another room.

A woman does not have to choose between her husband and her baby, but she may need to use discretion. It is no good raging against a man who feels like this. He cannot help it, and it is much better to get it out into the open.

'I have good firm breasts, and it may be selfish, but I don't want to spoil my figure.'

When a woman says this she is really talking about the delight that her partner takes in her breasts and is anxious that they will change, and with them, the relationship. The more unsure she is about the relationship the more she feels that any physical alteration will affect it. In fact, breast-feeding does not make breasts sag. Pregnancy involves glandular changes which may make breasts heavier and less firm. It is pregnancy which does this, not breastfeeding.

'*I don't feel confident that I shall ever know when the baby has had enough. It's all very well saying "let the baby guide you" but I'm not that sort of person. I want to be sure that it has taken the correct quantity.*'

A woman who feels like this may find bottle feeding much easier than breastfeeding, but it is probably still a good idea for her to try breastfeeding for at least a few weeks to see how it goes. She may discover unexpected pleasures and find that the baby is so obviously thriving that there is no question of not having enough milk.

On the whole, though, it is true that anyone who likes a very organized routine and who feels insecure outside a rigid framework of living will find breastfeeding anxiety-arousing. Having continuing emotional support from a breastfeeding counsellor who has herself breastfed may make all the difference.

So there is a case for bottle feeding for those who prefer it. Bottle feeding may also be necessary when a woman has to take certain kinds of medication which pass into her milk and could harm her baby. Most medicines are only present in breast milk in minute quantities and do not seem to cause any difficulty. Nearly always drugs given can be changed for a breastfeeding woman.

There is more about drugs in Chapter 13.

4. The breast

A woman's breast is a gland with connective tissues to support it and fat to protect it. It is one of the most important *exocrine* glands, that is, one which produces substances which are transported to other parts of the body. Such glands depend on hormones secreted by *endocrine* glands for their stimulation and development.

If a pregnant woman looks at her breasts in a mirror she will see that they have become larger and heavier than before the pregnancy started. The major part of this development takes place in the first months of pregnancy. A maternity bra bought just before you have your baby will still fit after birth. Although breast size changes between feeds, and they are largest just before the start of a feed, most of the growth has actually occurred long before this.

Immediately around the nipple is a circle of darker skin, the areola. This gets darker in pregnancy and lighter again after breastfeeding is finished. It is bumpy with *Montgomery's tubercles*, tiny raised glands ranged like the numbers on a clock, which become larger in pregnancy and may be one of the first signs that a woman has conceived. They secrete a fluid which keeps the nipple bathed and lubricated. When a mother has finished breastfeeding they return to their previous size and are barely noticeable.

The blood supply to the breast is much increased during pregnancy. Especially if you have fair skin you will notice that the blood vessels are much more obvious than formerly, the blue veins etched on the breast like an air photograph of a series of branching rivers and their tributaries.

Inside the breast there is a remarkable interconnecting network of passages and pools where the milk is manufactured and stored and through which it is ejected. There are fifteen to twenty clusters of *alveoli* or milk glands in each breast and the milk is produced within each grape-like lobule. There are little canals leading from the alveoli, called *ductules*, and larger ones, called *milk ducts*, down through which the milk travels, one for each bunch of alveoli, fifteen to twenty in all. Balloon-shaped sacs lying directly beneath the areola are *pools* from which the milk is pressed by the combined rhythmic action of the baby's tongue and jaws. Note that these are not in the nipple but that their upper ends are about level with the margin of the areola.

If the mother has a small areola the whole of it goes into the baby's mouth. Even if she has a larger one a portion of the areola must still be inside the mouth if the baby is to be able to draw the nipple in deeply.

The size of the breast does not matter and there is ample room for all these structures in small breasts. Just as people breathe equally well through a wide variety of noses, so women can breastfeed with very different sized and shaped breasts. A large-breasted woman should 'dimple' or hold the breast clear of the baby's nostrils, if necessary, so that he can breathe easily, or may prefer to hold him facing her with his legs under her arm.

HOW THE MILK IS MADE

Stimulation of the nipple by the baby's suckling, or even by thinking about it, sends messages to the hypothalamus. This produces a response in the pituitary gland at the base of the brain resulting in the release of the hormones prolactin and oxytocin. Prolactin travels in the blood stream to stimulate the alveoli to produce milk, which they synthesize from water, protein and lactose in the blood.

Oxytocin travels through the blood stream to the breast and stimulates the cells lining the alveoli to contract. This squeezes milk into the ducts, which contract and shoot the milk into the milk pools and from there down into the openings in the nipple, an action which is assisted and kept going by the baby's continued suckling. All this takes only a matter of seconds.

THE LET-DOWN REFLEX

A tingling, warm rush of blood into the breasts preparatory to the ejection of milk tells the mother that her breasts and the milk-making process are acting in response to her feelings about feeding her baby. The breasts actually get hotter when this occurs. 'Let-down' reflex is probably an unfortunate term as it suggests that the mother is depressed and the authors of one book on breastfeeding remind us that the mother is not 'let down' in the usual sense.[1] Some women never feel a powerful reflex, but still have plenty of milk and breastfeed happily. Some women do not like the feeling, and it is not uncommon for it to be experienced as uncomfortable or even painful in the first few days of breastfeeding especially if it is associated with uterine contractions which bring pain.

Women who do have a strong reflex are fortunate as they know that milk is about to stream from their breasts and are quite certain that the baby is being fed. In the beginning the reflex may not occur for a few *minutes* and then be felt strongly. This is a sure sign that it takes a little time for the process by which milk is made available to the baby to get started, and even if the baby is suckling *this preparatory time should not be counted as feeding*. Probably most women discover things that help the reflex get going, perhaps listening to music or simply visualizing the milk flowing.

Although the baby is only at one breast, the let-down reflex occurs in both and milk may actually spurt out from the other breast as well, so it is sensible to have a clean handkerchief or tissue ready to catch the jets from the other side if the mother finds this happens to her. Firmly holding the heel of the palm of a hand against the leaking breast will stop the flow.

PREPARING FOR BREASTFEEDING

A good deal of balderdash has been written about preparation of the breasts for nursing, almost invariably by men. Women are told to scrub their nipples with a nailbrush and toughen them up by rubbing them with alcohol. I cannot imagine a man agreeing to scrub his penis! The nipple is at least as sensitive as the penis, perhaps more so.

Any tissues which are hard tend to crack more readily. Lips hardened by wind and cold may crack too. Nipples, like lips, need to be soft, elastic and flexible. So if anything at all is used in preparation for breastfeeding it should be a cream or oil. Do not use anything scented in case this should prove an irritant. If you have allergies to wool and intend to use a cream containing lanolin, check first of all by doing a patch test over twenty-four hours on your inside elbow. If no redness appears, lanolin is all right for you.

In fact, neither cream nor oil is necessary, but it is a good idea to give the nipples airbaths or, if there is a chance, sun-baths, being careful not to burn them. Splash with water when you wash but do not use soap on them or try to scrape off any colostrum that has dried on the surface.

Nipples change shape during pregnancy and one that was flat or inverted may protrude well by the end of pregnancy, and stick out still more when the baby has been sucking for a bit. Women with small nipples can breastfeed. All that is required is that when the baby is put to the breast the nipple stands out from the surrounding tissue. A woman can tell if this is possible if she notices if her nipples project when she is cold or, perhaps more important, when she is sexually aroused when making love.

The nipple responds to emotions and gets ready for giving in the same way that the vagina changes its shape when she longs for her man to come in. This is why love-making which includes playing with the breasts and sucking and stimulating them is probably the best preparation for breastfeeding, and more natural and pleasurable than all the other manipulations, the rubbing, rolling and pulling in the bath, which are often suggested.

Love-making is also associated with the spontaneous release of oxytocin, which the French obstetrician Dr Michel Odent calls 'the happiness hormone',[2] and which is also responsible for the natural preparation during pregnancy of the breasts and nipples for breastfeeding and for milk ejection once the baby is born. Masters and Johnson[3] studied nipple erection in sexual excitement and discovered that when a woman was sexually aroused her nipples increased in length by 0·5 to 1·0 cm.

This is quite a different kind of experience from dutifully tugging at the nipples to try and make them change shape! In one study a group of pregnant women did nipple rolling for three weeks, but only on one nipple. They found there was no difference between the two nipples once their babies were born, and it did not appear to affect whether or not they became sore.[4]

True inverted nipples may be helped by wearing Woolwich shields (sometimes called Waller's shields after the doctor who invented them) under the bra for about ten to sixteen weeks at the end of pregnancy. There is no point in starting earlier than this. Glass ones are usually better than plastic because they press the nipple forward more firmly. They are obtainable on prescription or over the counter.

A Woolwich shield is not obvious to observers, although it may feel a little odd to someone who brushes against the woman. Some expectant mothers think it improves their shape, whereas others complain that they feel armour-plated. It may be more comfortable to wear for a few hours a day at first, and gradually to extend the time it is worn. Eventually the woman can, if she wishes, wear them at night too, but should not do this if they interfere with sleep. There is probably no additional advantage in wearing one for longer than six hours a day.

Some women find it difficult to prepare for breastfeeding because they dislike their breasts being touched by anyone and may not even like touching their breasts themselves. This may be because strong physical feelings of revulsion are aroused, or because erotic sensations are stimulated which for one reason or another then make the woman feel ashamed or even 'dirty'. I used to think that women who felt like this should not attempt to breastfeed, and always tried to give emotional support to any woman who has disclosed to me that this is how she feels. Almost invariably I have had to protect her from a group of expectant mothers in the childbirth education class which is enthusiastic about breast-feeding. I have since learned, however, that provided the woman is able to make her own free choice, and knows that her childbirth teacher, or whoever else discusses this with her, is able to accept happily whatever that choice is, she may well decide to try breastfeeding, and be very successful at it!

One woman told me that she could not bear to touch her own nipples because of the strong feelings this aroused so she did not think she could face the idea of breastfeeding. I agreed with her and said I thought she had made a sensible decision. I did point out that extraordinary changes some-times take place during pregnancy and that we may get to know our bodies, and like them, in new ways. Later in the pregnancy she told me she was finding that she could allow herself to touch her nipples a bit; we discussed how this felt. She could accept firm touch, but she could not bear a light, tickling touch. When she had her baby I was surprised to learn that she had started to breastfeed, that everything was going well and that she was enjoying it. She had had strong motivation to succeed by doing it all her own way, as she was still horrified at the thought of letting anyone else touch her breasts, and this included a midwife. I met her again much later and she told me she had had four more children and breastfed them all.

You will see that some books tell you that you ought to be expressing some colostrum in late pregnancy. I have known women become very anxious about this because they could not. They thought they must be doing something wrong or that there was nothing in their breasts and they would not be able to produce any milk. In some women colostrum seeps out readily and they find that it even stains underclothing. Others never see anything, except perhaps some slight mois-ture occasionally. Yet all these women can breastfeed. Nor is there any need to express colostrum in order to 'unplug the ducts' as women are sometimes told. The only advantage of expressing colostrum is that the expectant mother then knows that she can express, a skill which may come in useful after she has had the baby. She may also find it very reassuring to discover that the mammary glands are working and there is activity going on inside them. Colostrum is manufactured afresh by the breasts at the time of the baby's birth. You will not use it up if you express beforehand. If you would like to try it can be a good idea; if you do not have any inclination to express colostrum, leave it.

After the baby arrives the breastfeeding mother will want easily washed clothes that undo quickly at the front for feeding. Dresses with zips at the back are impossible. Blouses, T-shirts and sweaters with skirts, jeans and trousers make breastfeeding simple. When a new mother starts feeding she may not have the time to explore clothes shops, so it is useful to think ahead.

Breast pads are useful to tuck into the bra to prevent soiling of clothes. Disposable paper ones or a man's freshly laundered handkerchief are good, or one-way nappy liners or a one-way nappy cut up into rectangles is helpful in keeping clothing clean. Waterproof-lined pads keep the nipples too moist and should only be worn with evening clothes, silk, velvet or anything which one cannot risk staining with milk.

5. The momentous hour after birth

The baby takes the first breath and cries. The skin is suffused with pink. It moves against the mother's inner thighs. The mother can feel amazing life throbbing with energy against her own body, hears the primeval shout of a newborn human being and reaches out her arms to take her little, crumpled daughter. The baby's eyes are tightly closed, her mouth puckered, hair damp with tendrils curling over the deep curve of the nape of the neck, fine hairs like those on the skin of a peach cover her body with a silky bloom, hands are still wet and criss-crossed with lines from submersion in the uterine waters.

She comes to the mother's arms and is cradled against her skin. The lights are turned down. The baby's crying is stilled. There is quietness, for now one of the most important times in the life of a new human being is beginning to unfold.

In the hour that follows, whenever mother and baby can stay together in an environment where they can be in close physical contact in an atmosphere of love, extraordinary things begin to happen.

First the baby starts to relax. The struggle is over and she sinks more heavily against your body. You can feel the incredibly sweet warmth and weight of her as she becomes almost one with you again after the separation of delivery. Then she opens her eyes and looks straight at you. It brings a shock of delighted surprise. This is not just 'the baby'; here is a *person*. Aidan Macfarlane[1] says that in his taped transcripts one mother did not greet her baby till he opened his eyes, and then she said 'Hello' to him seven times in less than one and a half minutes!

This is as intense an experience for the father as it is for the mother. It is the first encounter.

The baby who is untrammeled by wrappings and is free to

make movements starts to discover self and the environment. Each hand begins to search the air. She touches her own face, for the first time moving in the medium of air rather than water. She encounters your skin. The actions are apparently aimless, like the movements of an anemone in a rock pool, but through them the baby is picking up signals. She is beginning, for the very first time, to learn the difference between space and solid objects, between hard and soft and rough and smooth, and even to start to differentiate between the 'me' and 'not me' which she will not fully understand until the end of the first year of life.

When her hands are not being used in this way they are curled into fists, but when they start on the intermittent task of discovering the environment they unfurl, open, and begin to scan with the efficiency of radar.

She turns her eyes towards your voice. It is as if she already knows it. She follows the movement of your hand. She gazes searchingly in your face.

The baby who is put straight in a crib after a few minutes, or who is left in her mother's arms, but encased in wrappings like a sausage, may be easy to handle but is unable to explore the world in this way. An avenue of discovery is closed and the unfolding first communication through the senses between the mother and her child is lost.

Once a baby is breathing well there can be no procedures which are more important than the need for mother, father and baby to get to know each other in their own time and in a setting which is comfortable, intimate and protected. Delivery of the placenta, weighing the baby and cleaning her up if necessary, cleaning and tidying the mother and moving her to another bed, a paediatric inspection, even champagne or cups of tea, can all take place later. If the placenta is not yet delivered the steady pressure of the baby's body nestled over the fundus is just enough to assist separation, combined with the suckling action of the baby and its effect on the uterus. Attendants can stand by and wait for the delivery of the placenta.

The baby's period of quiet alertness which usually follows delivery lasts for forty-five minutes to one hour.[2] The undrugged baby's eyes are wide open during part of this time and she responds to her environment and starts communicating with the mother through touch, eye contact and movements of her mouth associated with suckling. After that the baby tends to sink into a long sleep and may continue to be drowsy for several days. If the opportunity has not been used the mother should watch and wait for later alert states.

The experience in which both mother and baby begin to learn about each other is probably of much greater significance for human beings than the instant bonding which occurs between a goat and her kid or a cat and her kittens when the mother licks them. Human parents and their babies need time to introduce themselves to each other and develop a pattern of satisfying interaction. The synchronization which is beginning then takes place simultaneously at a number of physiological and sensory levels and develops into the 'in tune' communication described in Chapter 15.

THE BABY'S REFLEXES

The newborn bay has three feeding reflexes, inbuilt biological mechanisms which drive her to feed and to do so effectively. But they may be weakened or temporarily obliterated by analgesic or anaesthetic drugs which the mother had in labour and which have accumulated in the baby's blood stream.

One is the *rooting* reflex. If you watch carefully as you hold your baby close in the hour after birth you will see when she is ready to go to the breast because she will start to make mouth movements, opening and closing her mouth and twisting her lower jaw, and may turn her head from side to side as if hunting for something behind her ear. She may also screw up one eye at a time. If you touch her cheek (it does not matter which) she turns sharply from side to side and searches for the nipple in an urgent way with little, quick, darting movements.

The mother whose breasts are bare may find that her baby becomes obviously excited. It may be that she can smell her mother too. This is the moment to lean forward, lift her on to the nipple and to elicit the *sucking* reflex. The baby often enjoys first licking the nipple for a time. Then her mouth opens, the mother slips her nipple in and she starts to suck, at first perhaps rather experimentally, but later with growing confidence and *savoir faire*.

Although suckling is a reflex activity it is not as simple as the knee jerk reflex.

It is a highly complex, internally organized response, but it is also variable and able to take into account the nature of the external stimulation it encounters ... Sucking is, in fact, just one component of the total feeding act, which is made up of 'the rooting reflex' ... opening the mouth and grasping the nipple with the lips, sucking and swallowing. To function properly, these activities, together with breathing, must all be very finely integrated in sequence, so that together they make up a coordinated system that can deal effectively with a far from constant environment.[2]

Many new babies seem to have to learn how to keep on the nipple. If your baby drops off she will then root again unless she is sleepy. If you hold her with her cheek touching your breast your flesh itself acts as a stimulus to further searching for the nipple.

Some babies need encouragement to suck, especially premature babies and those still drugged from chemicals for pain relief received through the mother's blood stream. The best way to do this is to elicit the rooting reflex by again stroking the cheek or the side of her mouth.

It can be very tiring for a tiny premature baby to have to turn her head too, so it is important to support the head well. The easiest way to do this is to put a couple of pillows on the mother's lap and put the baby on her side facing the breast. The mother's arm rests on the pillow, curved along the baby's back, her hand cupping the buttocks.[3]

To obtain nourishment the baby needs to coordinate the sucking with the *swallowing* reflex. Only when the two are harmonized does true *suckling* take place. She has been sucking and swallowing while in the uterus and drinking the waters of her aquatic environment. She may also have been sucking her hand. When the mother feels quick localized movements which are obviously not a hand, knee or foot, it may be that the baby is rooting for a thumb or finger it has lost, for it can already suck for comfort in the uterus.

Some babies are eager to suckle from the moment they are born. Most take time to adjust to this startling new environment and are only ready to suckle after some twenty to thirty minutes. It is important that the mother who wants to put the baby to the breast after delivery realizes that her baby will tell her when he is ready and that to stuff a breast in his mouth before that moment is reached will produce disappointing results and possibly also a protesting baby.

There is no hurry. Simply hold the baby and watch him and the rooting reflex will announce the right time to offer him the breast. This can be difficult in some hospitals where pressure on the delivery suite means that nurses and midwives are anxious to get a mother 'processed' and out and the room cleaned up for the next delivery. Some progressive hospitals have instituted a system whereby mother, father and baby have extended time together in private to get to know each other immediately following delivery. It is worth asking at the hospital where you are thinking of having your baby whether parents and newborn can spend the first hour together. It is a very precious time and one important in the baby's life.

If the baby is wrapped in a towel or receiving blanket, undo this so that you have skin-to-skin contact. Hold her against your bare skin. The mother is a good source of heat after the work of the second stage of labour. Newborn babies can lose heat quickly and unless the room is very warm there should either be a heater or blanket over both mother and baby. Make sure that the hospital ventilation system is not streaming cold air over your baby. The greatest area of heat loss is the baby's head, so ensure that it is warm. The mother often feels cold and shaky after delivery and welcomes the additional warmth provided by electric heater or coverings.

The stimulus provided by the baby's suckling after delivery both contracts the tissues surrounding the alveoli to let down colostrum and releases oxytocin which contracts the mother's uterus. It may be experienced as an 'after pain'. It can be useful if the third stage is delayed and the placenta still undelivered. The placenta cannot contract and is thus peeled off the lining of the uterus and slips down into the vagina. Nowadays drugs are usually given to all women after delivery to ensure that this happens. But nature provides its own oxytocin if given a chance.[4] Suckling thus initiates a complex hormonal as well as behavioural bond.

If because of nursing routines or because the baby had to go to the nursery a mother is separated from him in the hour after birth she can create a similar meeting with her baby as soon as she can be alone with him and in flesh-to-flesh contact. When she is in hospital it is a good idea for her to pull the curtains round the bed, to undress herself and to unclothe her baby down to his nappy. She should make no attempt to put him to the breast at first, but simply lie him on her body and watch him. If he is past the particularly alert stage following delivery he may only stay awake and contented for a few minutes. When he indicates that he is ready to suckle she puts him to the breast. From then on she can observe her baby carefully to see when he is in the quiet, alert stage, and take every opportunity to let him find out about her and the world around him during these times. Both she and the baby can learn a surprising amount in times together like this.

6. The baby comes to the breast

The way in which the breast is given to the baby lays the pattern for future feeding and is often the decisive factor in whether or not it is a satisfying experience for the mother and child. But even if the first encounters have gone badly a fresh approach can be made, and a distressing experience turned into a happy one. It is not simply a matter of juxtaposing a breast and a baby, any more than love-making is just a matter of juxtaposing a vagina and a penis. With breastfeeding, as with all love relationships, it is not enough to love; we need to know how to *show* love. This is where the skills of breastfeeding can be important, especially if it does not seem to come naturally, and if because of what has occurred before, during the labour or because of being separated from each other in the immediate postpartum period, mother and baby start out at a disadvantage.

FIXING

After your baby is born you will want to put her to the breast. She will probably latch on eagerly and you will never think of exactly how it was done or why suckling is so simple. But some mothers and babies do not start off in the right way. Somehow the baby never seems to get at the correct angle or to get a good mouthful of breast, and the result is misery for both mother and baby.

Fixing is nothing to do with hard drugs. It is the art of getting the baby right on the nipple, instead of half on and dragging on it. It is vitally important because otherwise the mother tends to get sore nipples, the baby does not get sufficient milk, and the process of automatic milk manufacture is never triggered off. The technique of extracting the milk which is in the breast is essential for its further production.

The stimulus for both production and release of milk is the baby's suckling: demand creates supply.

If a woman is still in the first days of breastfeeding getting the baby fixed is probably the main thing she needs to bear in mind. Breastfeeding is a way of loving. Not getting the nipple deep into the baby's mouth is like never achieving penetration. The act is incomplete and the result is frustration for both mother and baby.

The easiest and most effective way of introducing the baby to the breast is to do so following delivery. This first encounter is then as if she has been born from your body only to come back to you cradled in your arms and drawing milk from your breast. The circle is completed.

If you are wearing a hospital gown your husband should untie it at the back and slip it down over your shoulders. There is an advantage in doing this even before delivery so that mother and baby can have skin contact from the beginning. When the newborn begins to root for the nipple or to make sucking movements with her mouth, and not before, offer the breast.

The woman who has had pain-relieving drugs which have dulled her mind or a long, tiring labour may welcome help in supporting the baby. It is difficult to feel secure on the usual narrow delivery table in hospital. The husband can prop his wife well up and hold her in his arms as she holds the baby or can put one arm round her with the other supporting arm round the baby. The baby's head should lie in the crook of her elbow.

Some babies seem to be searching for the nipple but do not realize what it is for even when they have found it. Most lick it before they latch on ready for suckling. The baby who continues to explore the nipple with the tongue will get further interested if a drop or two of colostrum is expressed. This is something that a man can also do for his wife. Either the mother or the father can then gently 'tease' the baby with the nipple, touching it lightly against her cheeks and each side of the mouth. If the baby is ready to suckle she will open her mouth and the nipple can be introduced.

When you slip the nipple into the baby's searching mouth

make sure that she can get a satisfying mouthful. There are special touch receptors deep in the mouth, stimulation of which gives the baby pleasure and ensures that the right suckling action is initiated. Chloe Fisher, a midwife tutor in Oxford, who has had vast experience with helping new mothers start breastfeeding, believes that every breastfeeding problem stems from not getting the baby on in the first place. She sometimes meets mothers who have persevered with breastfeeding for weeks and weeks, albeit in a very unsatisfactory way, and who have, she says, 'suffered ghastly traumas', whose difficulties derive from never having managed to get the baby fixed on the breast.

Sore nipples, mastitis, an inadequate milk supply and an under-fed baby are all consequences of failing to get the baby fixed. Even a woman who had a great deal of milk to start with and a dramatic let-down reflex may find that her milk disappears unless she is able to get the baby right on. This is because a powerful let-down reflex with initial spurts of milk which are projected into the baby's mouth without him needing to do any active suckling can lead a woman into thinking that her baby is well on the breast when in fact he is not. When the first milk ejection is finished the baby is then no longer able to get milk and starts to fuss and struggle, or drops off the nipple after having had only very little milk.

Only when the nipple is drawn into the back of the mouth can the baby suckle effectively. Suckling is not the same as sucking. A baby does not suck in the same way as we might suck a milk shake or a cocktail through a straw. If she did so a partial vacuum would be created and very little milk would actually get into her mouth. Instead the baby uses a strong jaw movement. If you watch you will see the muscles above the ears working hard. This is why dentists say that breastfeeding assists the normal development of the jaw and teeth, and why it is sometimes claimed that breastfeeding helps the development of good, clear speech.

If you put the tip of a finger in your mouth and suck it the action is equivalent to sucking through a straw. But if you take the joint at the base of your thumb, drawing it in with suction (and because you have teeth lifting them up off the flesh) you will get an action involving the whole jaw which is more like that used by a baby at the breast.

The baby also uses her tongue pressed against the underside of the nipple to squeeze out milk. So it is important that the tongue is *under* the nipple. This squeezing is done with the strong central part of the tongue, not with its tip. (Young children often have a good deal of difficulty in learning to pronounce 'th' and some other sounds involving the tip of the tongue.) This is another reason why the nipple must be well in the baby's mouth.

When the nipple and areola are not between the baby's jaws the milk cannot flow so easily. But it is not only a question of a reduced milk supply. The mother is also likely to get a sore nipple because the baby tends to chew and drag on it where the nipple meets the breast. It is understandable that if a woman is feeling nervous about breastfeeding, rather frightened of this angry, extraordinarily vigorous baby, anxious that she may not succeed, inhibited about putting on a performance in front of a helper, or even, as can happen, if she feels that breastfeeding is physically distasteful, she draws back on offering the nipple so that the baby then grips the junction between nipple and areola, where a sore is most likely to develop. Once she has a sore a vicious circle is created, because then it takes nerves of steel to deliberately introduce the nipple in a generous way into the baby's mouth.

Though many expectant mothers are concerned that their nipples may be too flat, short nipples are often just right. A woman with long nipples, on the other hand, may encounter difficulties because she cannot easily get a good part of the areola into the new baby's mouth. There is an enormous statue of 'Maternity' outside a hospital in Mexico City which depicts a mother drawing her child to her bosom. Her nipples are like Bologna sausages and I fear feeding was not likely to be a success because the baby would have found it impossible to get those huge nipples into the back of its mouth. Fortunately the pair were frozen in immobility and the maternal breasts were never put to the test!

COMFORTABLE POSITIONS FOR FEEDING

All this makes it sound technically very complicated. In fact,
if the mother holds the baby so that his cheek is against her
breast and his legs tucked under her arm on the opposite
side it is easy to get into a good position. She lifts her breast
into her baby's mouth and cuddles him close. Sometimes,
especially with a tiny newborn, it is easier if she puts a pillow
on her lap and rests the baby on this. An alternative position is to place the baby with his legs under her arm and his
head facing her, supporting it with her hand. It is usually
simplest to have the baby lying on a pillow if you prefer this
position.

It is probably best to experiment with positioning the
baby in privacy where you can make mistakes without feeling
grossly incompetent. It is also important to see that you are
sitting comfortably yourself, not on the edge of a chair as if
waiting for the next train on platform three but sitting well
back with head and shoulders supported by cushions.

In the early days this is simpler than it sounds. A woman
who has had an episiotomy and stitches is likely to feel that
she is sitting on thorns. She needs to get on to one buttock
or the other or lean back so that there is no pressure on the
site of the suturing. Pillows and a rubber ring to sit on can
help. Even a rubber ring which children have at the seaside
can be satisfactory. Either way, with a tender bottom, a baby
to put to the breast and a nipple to get into the baby, it can
seem like a juggling act.

Some nurses on postnatal wards insist that mothers must
sit on chairs to feed. Some say that they have to get back
into bed. This is a pity, because the essential thing is that a
woman does what feels most comfortable for her.

A mother who has had a Caesarean birth will find it painful
to lie with the baby across her abdomen. It is better to lie on
one side, with the elbow propped up, Roman-style, and the
baby beside her on the bed, or to sit up with the baby facing
her and his legs tucked under her arm.

In your own home you may choose to be nestled into a
polystyrene foam-filled bean bag, which can be ideal for nurs-

ing, half reclining against a pile of big cushions on the floor
or bed, sitting in a rocking chair, on a settee or easy chair,
propped against a tree in the garden, lying on your side on
the hearthrug in front of a log fire, or even swinging in a
hammock or propped in a warm bath. (Make sure the room is
well heated for this so that the baby does not get chilled.) If
there are strict rules in hospital a woman can still relax and
do it her way when she gets home.

In different cultures there is a wide variety of preferred
positions for breastfeeding. There is certainly no one 'right'
way. In some African societies a mother can even feed her
baby while it is still on her back by flinging her elongated
breast over her shoulder! So there are no rules, and it is
worth experimenting, even if you may not choose to do the
latter.

When the baby is lying on the mother's lap, it is probably
easiest to position the baby's head so that it is in the crook of
her arm. She should use a movement of her whole arm to
guide the baby to the breast or to reposition him. This is why
relaxed shoulders are important. It is impossible to move
freely and smoothly with tense shoulders and stiff arms.

THE ART OF 'TEASING'

Chloe Fisher says that a baby who has never been coaxed and
'teased' enough with the inviting nipple may never open her
mouth sufficiently to get a good grasp on the breast, so that
true suckling does not get a chance to start. 'Thrusting the
breast into the baby's mouth is fatal,' she warns, 'because
this alters the shape of the areola and can be distressing for
the baby.' This is why help sometimes offered by nurses who
grip the front of the breast, pressing on their thumb and fore-
finger as if they were thrusting a *petit four* into the baby's
mouth may apparently work, because at least the baby *looks*
as if he is feeding, but is unlikely to get him fixed in the right
way. What often happens is that the mother draws back because her breast is tender and this hurts, while the baby
gets only the nipple and the outer breast tissue immediately
surrounding it, not the underlying glandular structures which

contain the canals through which milk must be pressed in order for it to flow into his mouth.

I have often seen mothers holding back so that they can manipulate the baby's head with their hands and 'plug' it in more firmly. Babies fight this and get confused because when anyone touches their cheeks or the sides of their heads they respond by rooting and turn the head from side to side in search of the nipple. The mother, however, wants her baby to turn *towards* her only. She applies firmer pressure from her fingers at both sides of the baby's head, sometimes gripping it in a vice, and the baby continues struggling to turn from side to side. The mother may be lucky enough to pop the nipple in and the baby accepts it with glad surprise, but all too often something like a fight starts and the contest ends in misery for both.

With a baby who has not yet quite caught on to what it is all about seduction and gentle persuasion are better than determined efforts at pushing and shoving the baby's head against the nipple. After all, taking an analogy from sex, a woman may not enjoy a man merely thrusting against her and might prefer a more subtle approach with light stroking in the right place. The mother may have to find the right place to stimulate her baby to seek the nipple, and as we have seen this is likely to be at either side of the mouth. Touch at either side will stimulate the baby to turn *both* ways. She may also have to discover what kind of touch is most effective. This is part of what it is to embark on an intimate relationship with a new human being, for which there is no recipe for success, only the loving interaction between a mother and baby.

7. The hospital

In maternity hospitals today mothers are more likely than ever before to have the opportunity of rooming-in and to find that breastfeeding is encouraged and demand-feeding the accepted policy. That is a terrific advance over the system as it used to be even a few years ago. There has been a breakthrough in baby feeding and in recognition of the importance of the mother and baby being able to function as a dyadic unit, a nursing couple.

But having said that, let us take a closer look at what is actually happening in hospitals. There is sometimes a gulf between theory and practice. It is worth inquiring about the hospital where you plan to have a baby exactly what occurs at ward level, and finding out, both from inquiry of the hospital and from women who have had babies in it recently, the environment which is likely to be provided for you to start off your life with your baby. If you do not like what is provided, you may prefer to change the hospital, or to arrange for early discharge home to the care of the community midwife, or to have a home delivery. For at home you can 'do your own thing', with expert guidance and support when you need it, from a midwife who comes in as your guest rather than as someone who controls the postnatal environment in every aspect. It is very much easier to arrange for this in advance than to decide during your postpartum stay that you cannot endure the hospital any longer and that you must leave.

Some hospitals are very happy places and mothers look back on their stay with pleasure. I remember one woman describing a huge London teaching hospital as 'a sanctuary'. Others are not, and I believe are just about the last place a new mother and her baby should be. What suits one person may not appeal to you. The important thing is to investigate and to take an active part in creating the kind of environment in which you would like to be in the first days after the birth. Once in hospital it is up to you to decide whether you try as far as possible to determine your own course of action, or whether this will result in such unnecessary stress that it is better to wait to start to do things as you want them when you get home. *Only you can judge* the situation at the time and the state of your own feelings. Whatever you choose to do there is no need to feel guilty because you did not do the opposite! If you came to the conclusion that it was best to 'go with the stream' while in hospital and were not happy with the way breastfeeding was started, it is a good idea to treat your first day home as day one. Keep the baby in bed with you or close beside your bed, and suckle whenever she opens her eyes or attracts your attention by crying or fussing.

In most British hospitals nowadays the baby is handed to the mother after delivery and she is able to suckle on the delivery bed. There is no need to *ask* to do this. The baby is yours. If you have a hospital gown which does up at the back ask your husband or other labour companion to undo it at the top so you can slip it over your shoulder. Some hospitals have a rule that the first feed a baby receives must be glucose water or sterile water. The colostrum that is already in your breasts is very much better for the baby than either of these. You may be willing to compromise and let the hospital give its test feed *after* you have put your baby to the breast. If this compromise is unacceptable to you ask if you can talk to the paediatrician.

It is sad that in some hospitals today, even when there is a token (or even sometimes genuinely enthusiastic) encouragement for breastfeeding, mothers are still implicitly taught to doubt their own capacity for producing milk and for relating to the baby in a mutually satisfying way. The baby is tucked up neatly in a cot when it would be much better for both baby and mother if it were being cuddled and kissed and explored and could lie beside its mother in her bed close to her warm body.

In my own study of women's experiences in some 300 hospitals in the United Kingdom, based on detailed letters from close on 1,800 women who had had babies in 1977 and the first months of 1978,[1] and further information provided by the Senior or Divisional Nursing Officer for Midwifery, it emerged that mothers were often dissuaded from handling their babies, because it was not considered 'good' for them, ('you won't have time to do it at home', and 'you'll spoil him') that handling time was sometimes strictly limited to the half hour or so allowed for feeds, ('We were told to feed, change and put them down in half an hour at most', said one mother) and that in a great many hospitals babies were not permitted on their mothers' beds, let alone in them. A mother who wanted to go to sleep with her hand still in the baby's cot said she was told to 'stop messing with the baby'. I cannot forget one letter, from a woman who had lost a baby with a cot death, and had then followed this with a tubal pregnancy. At last she was pregnant for the third time and her baby was born. She lifted her two-day-old daughter out of her cot 'just to look at her and hold her', when the Sister, in front of the other mothers in the ward, said, 'That's another spoiled brat in the making.'

In spite of publicity about the desirability of breastfeeding and the risks of bottle feeding, babies in some hospitals are still routinely being given bottles in the nursery: 'As the breastmilk is not properly "in" the first few days they fill them up with bottles just to keep them quiet . . . I tried (to breastfeed) for three days and gave up . . . I still feel bitter about this.' Mothers wrote of being laughed at when they were anxious to go to their babies in special care baby units and asked that they should not be given bottles. One wrote that the Sister had told her that she had never heard of a baby rejecting the breast because it had got used to the bottle, and the mother added that she could have told her all about it, as this was just what her previous baby did.

Many hospitals changed to a system of modified demand-feeding during 1977 and 1978. But even when a system is described by the administration as one of 'demand-feeding' ward activities are often still organized on the assumption that feeds take place four-hourly, from 6 a.m. on, there is often a proviso that a baby must not be allowed to sleep longer than five hours and must not be fed more frequently than every three hours (or in some hospitals two) and women are not allowed to feed during visiting, rest and meal-times, when the ward is being cleaned and during doctors' rounds, which leaves only certain very restricted times when they *can* feed. As one head of midwifery wrote: 'Feeding on demand is encouraged but in practice this works out as scheduled feeding.' A leaflet, intended for nursery nurses, sent me by the Divisional Nursing Officer of another hospital which practises 'demand-feeding', states that 'feeds should be arranged so that mothers go to the dining-room promptly for meals at mid-day and 6 p.m.', and that the baby should be 'fed and down in its cot again within five hours of the previous feed'. In yet another hospital which has changed to a demand-feeding routine 'procedures like weighing and bathing were timed to be just before feed-time', but the feed-time in theory, at any rate, no longer existed. One mother wrote that 'at the traditional hours of 10, 2, 6, and 10 the drinks trolley of water and bottles for the bottle feeders would arrive, and a nurse would suggest that we feed our babies now'. Her baby had often been fed and was sleeping when he was supposed to be weighed: 'I had to say loudly and firmly "I'm demand-feeding" when at the traditional feed-times my child was asleep.'

Mothers frequently wrote that it was demand-feeding 'compatible with ward routines', or 'at convenient times for the staff', or 'so long as it does not interfere with the running of the ward'. Many women accepted this as inevitable. In most of the hospitals which women described this 'demand-feeding' was not instituted until the third day or the milk had come in, or as one Senior Nursing Officer wrote, 'from the third or fourth day when we are satisfied that the nipples are satisfactory'. It is as if each woman had to pass a test of milk production and nipple normalcy before she was allowed to feed her baby when it cried.

There was hardly a hospital which did not limit sucking time with the intention of saving the mother's nipples, the mother being told to take the baby off after two minutes at first, then three minutes the next day and so on, regardless often of whether the baby had actually been sucking, whether the woman had experienced a let-down reflex which would have released milk to make it available for the baby, and therefore of whether the baby had been successful in getting any milk at all. Mothers were often instructed to wash their nipples before picking up the baby, so turning the feed into a ritualized hygienic technique, and in many hospitals had to go to the nursery to feed or sit up in a chair rather than lie or sit in bed.

In some hospitals which have a fairly flexible approach feeding routines may be adjusted to nurses' hours of duty rather than to babies' needs: 'I was asked to feed the baby one evening during visiting so that my nurse could go off duty. This meant my husband leaving early' (because in this hospital husbands are not allowed to be present during breastfeeds).

Some hospitals had adopted the system of handing mothers charts on which they filled in the length of sucking times and their own observations on the baby. But old attitudes die hard and as one mother said: 'I felt inhibited about owning up to each nibble of colostrum' and others said that they 'cheated' when filling them in. In a Scottish hospital which had adopted this system a mother said that she was 'scolded for too frequent feeds. I continued to do so, but filled in the feed chart wrong, so we were all happy.'

Authoritarian attitudes do not disappear overnight unfortunately. In one hospital in which there is a 'demand-feeding' policy babies are supposed to be back in their cots following feeds. 'No time for cuddles', one mother commented, 'and I didn't feel the baby was mine until I took her home', and one mother said that a nurse said ' "Stop playing with your baby and feed her" – which is what I was trying to do'. New mothers seem very vulnerable to these authoritarian attitudes.

In another hospital a woman asked to be woken at night to breastfeed, but was not and says she was told that glucose had been given instead. She was disappointed at the time, but in looking back on it later she was shocked that she did not protest. She said: 'I'm amazed at the way I am taken over by institutional care, thirty-seven years old, mother for the fourth time, teaching a large class of juniors up to a month before the birth. I couldn't assert myself, submitted to a general telling off for smoking in the bathroom though I don't smoke, even being ordered to put away my rainbow Kleenex, a gift from my youngest daughter, off my locker before visitors arrived.'

If you do not act with the confidence and *savoir faire* which you feel you *ought* to have, do not think you are alone in this; other women have done just the same.

In many of these hospitals mothers described members of staff as 'enthusiastic' about breastfeeding and midwives and nurses often demonstrated remarkable patience in helping women to breastfeed. They wanted to help, but they often did not know how to. Sometimes the assistance they provided proved distressing for the mother. This happened, for example, when a nurse grabbed the mother's engorged breast and pummelled or crammed a sore nipple and areola into the baby's mouth (one mother was highly critical of 'well-meaning nurses hauling my boobs about'), or when a baby was slow to suck and, as one mother said, 'The nurse kept flicking her and smacking her, then pushing her on to my breast. I felt as if my baby was not mine.' Often, too, nurses did not have the knack of instilling confidence: 'The midwife asked me if I wanted to breastfeed and when I said I did she told me my nipples were flat.' 'If you get sore nipples you'll probably have to give up', said one nurse as she wheeled away a crying baby.

The high incidence of jaundice associated with induction of labour, especially when epidural anaesthesia is used too,[2] means that in some hospitals jaundiced babies are given water by bottle every two hours. Mothers in these hospitals sometimes encountered difficulties in breastfeeding. 'We sobbed our hearts out,' wrote one woman, 'because they hadn't the thirst to feed from our breasts.' This woman, whose baby was only slightly jaundiced, did not give the water and lactation improved as her baby sucked.

Some hospitals give all newborn babies a feed of glucose water within an hour of birth, and some offer this regularly until the breast milk comes in, the idea being initially to discover if the baby is swallowing without difficulty and that in this way it can be ensured that no baby is likely to get hypoglycaemic, with resulting mental retardation. There is a case for this with very small babies whose growth in the uterus is inadequate, and also for the babies of diabetic mothers, but there is no reasonable case for doing this to all babies, regardless. Yet this is what is happening in our hospitals. Normal babies do not require extra sugar. What they do need is their mothers' colostrum.

It is the practice in many hospitals to routinely separate mother and baby for anything from a few hours to a day or so, and to tell the mother that she needs rest. The mother was sometimes told that this was because the baby must be in a specially warm nursery at this time. A mother whose baby was separated from her in a nursery at eighty degrees plus remarked, 'I wonder how the human race survives in countries where the temperature is lower than this?' The work of Klaus and Kennell[3] has demonstrated that this is an important time in the developing interaction between mother and baby, and even women who had no theories about this and had not read the recent psychological literature often said they could not rest and lay longing for their babies. This longing to touch, hold and explore the baby is a dynamic factor in establishing breastfeeding, and it seems a pity that it is neglected and ignored in so many hospitals. It is also disturbing that in some hospitals (and it appears to be particularly those in which a special care baby unit is on the same floor as delivery rooms) a proportion of babies are still being sent to special care for no reason which is apparent or explained to the mother. One mother remarked that it was the quickest and easiest thing to do with a baby born at night as it avoided disturbing patients on the postnatal wards. As a result mothers are separated from their babies for even longer periods than when the baby is simply taken to the ward nursery.

Staff on night duty in hospitals often believe that it is important for new mothers to get 'a good night's sleep' and failed to wake them, even when they have asked to be roused, to give their babies a night feed. This is distressing for a mother who does not want her baby to be given any cow's milk at all, however modified to make it more suitable for human babies, and means that she is deprived of the stimulus provided by suckling for increased milk production. All too often, it is a vicious circle, with the baby given a bottle feed so that the mother can rest, and this resulting in her milk supply never building up because the physiological stimulus has been omitted and feeds skipped. Occasionally staff seem to be misinformed about the mechanisms of lactation. In at least one hospital mothers are taught how to make up bottle feeds so that their breasts can 'charge up' overnight.

Mothers often remark that the hospital staff's only interest was in the baby's weight gain and that this led to test-weighing before and after feeds which made them tense and anxious about not producing enough. When a baby was discovered to have lost weight, or not regained its birth weight by the day laid down as the target by the paediatrician, recourse was had to the bottle as the only solution. Test weigh- was also used unwisely for one feed only on, for example, the first and fifth days of life. Babies, like adults, take different quantities at different times, and this is a pretty pointless exercise, which seems almost calculated to worry mothers.

In some hospitals feeds are still strictly timed and the baby is given a 'topping-up' bottle of formula if it has not finished 'on time'. If a baby was sleepy this reduced each feed to a tussle as the mother tried to wake her child sufficiently to suck and to keep him at it.

A hospital administration sent me a booklet which stated: 'One of the most important routines is baby feeding; this does not mean that there is no feeding between regular times, but the establishment of a regular routine is preferable.' Success in breastfeeding quite clearly in the eyes of staff in this hospital consists in achieving a timetable. Mothers are warned not to 'over-handle' their babies: 'We were not allowed to comfort the baby by cuddling it, even though it was alongside us', and women are told not to carry the baby 'in case you drop it'.

In another large hospital mothers are told that feeding is

scheduled because staff cannot assist except at set times and one mother who had her baby there wrote: 'No wonder difficulties arise. Babies are often woken to be fed when they are not hungry, and left to scream for half an hour or so while worried mums could only stand by helpless.'

Some hospitals still routinely provide topping-up bottles of formula after every breastfeed, and mothers may have no choice about whether to offer these to their babies. A mother wrote: 'I felt like a very naughty schoolgirl when I returned an almost full bottle to the nursery one day, having spent an hour trying to force-feed Katrina, to be turned back to try again because she'd be "screaming for food in another hour".'

One of the commonest complaints from mothers was that they are given often unsolicited and conflicting advice from nurses and others who were eager to help but who had no common policy about coping with breastfeeding problems and often very little practical experience of it. I believe that it is virtually impossible to give a mother help until you have sat quietly with her and watched her and the baby together to see what is happening between them. The counsellor can then help the mother analyse the interaction for herself and discover the main themes. It is a bit like discussing the theme of a poem or a novel; you cannot do this with any honesty until you have read it carefully. It is amazing how would-be advisors give instructions about breastfeeding which are irrelevant to the needs of that particular mother and that particular baby. The conflicting advice confuses mothers, who try first one thing and then another, and so indirectly it may confuse the baby too. It seems the ideal prescription to result in failure to breastfeed.

Women also wrote that they were expected to take sleeping pills 'dished out like Smarties', one mother said, and other drugs against pain. One woman said staff provided these four times a day. They were concerned to produce uncontaminated milk for their babies and were frightened of sleeping through and failing to wake to breastfeed the baby. In some hospitals there was no chance of avoiding this kind of medication, and it contributed to women's anxiety about breastfeeding.

Rigid ward routines are incompatible with demand-feeding and in some hospitals where demand-feeding has been instituted there seems to be a continual conflict between the needs of babies and the priorities of ward administration. Babies had to be in their cots or in the nursery before any visitors were allowed in; every extraneous or disorderly thing was swept off the top of the woman's locker; crying babies were wheeled out of earshot; mothers must be back in bed looking neat and tidy. Meals must be eaten on time or the dinner ladies get upset and there is no question of keeping a meal hot for the mother who happens to be breastfeeding at the time. Many mothers found it difficult to learn to observe and respond to their baby's signals in a sensitive way in such an atmosphere.

But perhaps even more counter-productive in terms of breastfeeding is the apparent relegation of the mother into the role of 'patient', an object on whom the hospital staff act for her own good. She then either finds herself fighting the system or becoming passive and institutionalized within a few hours of admission. In many hospitals it is clear that new mothers are encouraged to become dependent and are not allowed to make any meaningful decisions about their babies while they are still inside the hospital. One mother said, 'Sister said she had been expecting trouble from me because I was one of those mothers who is determined to breastfeed come what may'; 'He belonged to the hospital until day ten and that was it.' 'The nurses were liable to take the baby away with no explanation and were surprised when asked what they were about to do! ... For those (mothers) who failed to follow the rules a good "telling off" was expected.' 'I felt that I was one of the cogs in a machine and not a person at all. Until I got my baby home I had not really had that much contact with him at all.' Another woman who said she was not permitted to make the simplest decisions about her baby became very depressed with 'a hopeless feeling of inadequacy' which she attributed to the depersonalization resulting from hospital care. Even if a woman manages to start to breastfeed under these conditions she is very likely to lose her nerve when she is catapulted out of the hospital and has to start taking decisions about the baby on her own at home. A woman whose baby was kept in the nursery for three days and brought to her only for feeds, and after that 'one graduated to collecting babies at feed time, then to changing them after a feed, then to giving a bath on the seventh day', said she could not 'accept' her baby, 'except in a rather abstract way', and was 'nervous of handling her'; 'I was in no position to take decisions over her care ... Once I got home the contrast was a shock; suddenly complete responsibility was on me, and I felt on edge constantly.' She wrote when her baby was nearly a year old and said: 'The experience haunts me still.'

Mothers are often still discharged from hospital with free bottles of formula and a selection of little packets 'just in case', and powerful commercial interests, supported by the National Health Service, persuade the new mother, who especially with her first baby is almost by definition lacking in confidence, that she may have insufficient breast milk and her baby ought to be given the benefit of this or that milk formula.

The new concern for discovering potential baby-batterers shortly after their babies are born also distresses some mothers who are slow in feeling spontaneous love for their newborn. Not all women fall in love with their babies at first sight, and yet tenderness, compassion, and later often passionate love grow through the first days and weeks after delivery, and are better able to do so if the environment is one in which the mother feels relaxed and cherished herself. Some women are aware that they are being watched to see if they handle the baby as a loving mother should, make the correct expressions of delight and 'bond' satisfactorily in the eyes of the nursing staff. 'They don't like anything except 100 per cent concentration on the job', one mother remarked. She wanted to watch a TV programme while she was breast-feeding. 'The suggestion that I minded more about the 10,000 metres was tantamount to baby battering.' Another mother, whose baby was partially paralysed, felt that the child was continually 'thrust' at her to attempt to breast-feed because they thought she was in danger of rejecting it.

She felt under such pressure to love this 'helpless, unresponsive baby' and it was so 'emotionally draining' that she
avoided going to the special care baby unit except when she
had to, and may have been more at risk of rejecting her baby
because of staff anxiety that she was not accepting it as they
thought she should. This raises many interesting questions
about the effects of unskilled and insensitive 'baby-batterer
watching'.

It can also be very difficult emotionally for a breastfeeding
mother in the rush and bustle of a busy hospital ward. Most
hospitals are ill adapted to fostering the subtle and important
relationship which is developing between mother and baby.
Very few mothers felt they had a rest in hospital, and those
who did were often in wards where babies were kept mostly
in the nurseries. A hospital ward, however partitioned and
even if constructed for the convenience of nursing staff on
the race-track principle (a name which itself suggests a
desperate endeavour to catch up with time) or divided into
four bed wards, is rarely conducive to relaxation after having
a baby. 'There were so many do's and don'ts, not only about
baby care, but little regulations about how much you could
have on your bedside locker, when you could sit in the
lounge ... We didn't find out we were in someone's bad
books until after we had committed our crime.'

A large proportion of the women who wrote said they were
tired, exhausted, confused, bewildered or 'worn out'. Some
said they felt 'regimented' and were only too glad to get
home for a rest and a chance to enjoy their babies in their
own time in peace. There were references to 'conveyor belts'
and 'factory systems', 'a constant stream of changing faces',
'a general racket ... like Piccadilly Circus', and many women
felt alienated from their own babies; 'It was an environment
in which it is difficult for mother and baby to get to know
each other.'

In hospitals like this one must conclude that women
breastfeed *in spite of* rather than because of the care available!

Some hospitals are very different. There are some splendid
lactation sisters around and nurses who have made a special

study of breastfeeding and give willing, sensitive and skilled help. But you cannot *expect* this quality of care and if you encounter it it means that you are, by chance or design, in an exceptional hospital. I believe that we should make our hospitals the kind of places we want them to be, to provide a warm, loving environment in which not only a baby is delivered, but a new family is born. This can only happen when we are brave enough to ask questions and discover what is going on behind their walls. It can only happen, too, when we keep open a possible alternative to hospital, and are able to decide, if we wish, to go home, or even perhaps never leave it, and start the breastfeeding experience in the familiar and comforting setting of our own bedrooms.

If you have difficulties with breastfeeding your local community midwife will often be able to help you. Many community midwives specialize in helping breastfeeding mothers. The expert help of a community midwife tends to be undervalued today compared with the technological expertise of nurses and midwives working in 'high risk' units who concentrate on the detection of pathological factors. But the midwife who works for at least part of the time *outside* the hospital, in the community, is the person most likely to understand how to support a physiological, natural process.

8. The baby

Babies have had different experiences in the uterus. They pass through different kinds of birth experiences. And they have personalities. Before you have a baby they may look like so many bundles in cots, all rather squashed, some dark, some fair, some large, some small, but without much to distinguish one from another. After you have the baby you realize that all babies are different, and that yours is unique. You are quite right. Take with a pinch of salt all advice you are given about 'the' baby. The only relevant help must apply to you and *your* baby.

For some babies the uterus has been a comfortable place where they obtained good nourishment and all needs were automatically met as they rocked in the cradle of their mothers' bodies. But for others we can be certain that it did not correspond to our adult fantasies about the uterus as a safe haven to which we long to return, and that it failed to nourish the baby adequately. We now know that it is not a completely peaceful, utterly dark place unaffected by what is going on outside it, and that bright light filters through, that babies are affected by maternal physiological and intense emotional states and respond to sounds going on outside, including music (notice what happens at a concert when the cymbals clash), people's voices at certain pitches, loud machinery and the disturbing, penetrating but short-lived invasion of diagnostic ultra-sound.

Babies are also affected in one way or another by their journey into the world. For some it is difficult, for others fairly easy. Birth can be a strenuous business for some. The undrugged baby is not a passive bundle but makes strong reflex movements which help its progress down the birth canal. However straightforward the labour, being born must feel like being cast up on the shore after having been tossed for several hours in a stormy sea. Often then, too, instead of welcoming arms to quieten and soothe and a mother's warm, soft breast to nestle against, the baby is assailed with bright lights and loud noises and is handled as if it were a piece of meat being packaged for the supermarket.

Frederick Leboyer[1] has focused in the style of a poet on the often brutal way in which we treat our newborn babies. They are no mere bundles of flesh but exquisitely sentient beings. They are travellers who have already come on a long journey, across the little space of nine inches from the uterus to the world outside their mothers' bodies.

Babies are also affected by drugs the mother has received in labour. These chemical substances change the newborn baby's behaviour for days and even sometimes weeks after birth. They are likely to have their greatest effect just when a woman is starting to breastfeed, and it is therefore important to know how a baby may be affected so that you can understand the situation and adapt your own behaviour to handle it.

The simplest way of looking at the baby's state of well-being after delivery is to study the Apgar rating. This is a straightforward test of neuromuscular response and activity in the newborn developed by an American woman doctor, which anybody observant can do. It is usually assessed at one minute after birth and again at 5 minutes. We start exams very early these days! 10 is full marks, and most babies get 7 and up at delivery. A baby gets 2 if the heart rate is more than 100, 2 if it is breathing well, 2 if it is pink all over, 2 if it is making strong movements, and 2 if a catheter put into a nostril makes it sneeze or splutter, half marks for each of these categories if it cannot meet these standards. Even if a baby starts off with a fairly low mark it usually has something over 7 by the second assessment.

The Apgar rating is a very rudimentary test which codifies observations that midwives, and peasant midwives too, who have never filled in a form or seen a chart, have known all along. It does not take much expertise to realize that if a baby is not breathing, and it is limp and grey, and does not react when you handle it, it is in a bad way! (If the heart was beating, but slowly, this baby, in desperate need of resuscitation, would score an Apgar 1.) It provides a rough and ready record of how a baby is immediately after delivery, however, and this may be useful in assessing the baby's needs later. Babies who did not have an easy start to life may need special care, and sometimes perplexing and difficult behaviour in the days and weeks afterwards can be related to a difficult beginning. You cannot change your baby's experience of birth in retrospect, but you can help her feel safe and loved; the newborn who has been through this shattering experience may benefit from having a special closeness and security.

Primal therapy[2] teaches that birth is for all of us a dramatic and important experience and moulds our characters in ways of which we are usually oblivious. Therapists claim that when birth has been hard, as adults we need to relive the experience through re-enacting it in the company of others who can receive us in safety.

The parents of a baby who has had such a traumatic entry into the world need not wait for this, but can immediately offer an environment specially adapted to her needs. The basis is careful observation of what seems to make the baby feel good, and reduction of stress to a minimum. A baby who hates his nappy being changed still needs changing, of course, but it should be done in an unhurried way, with as few movements as possible, while you talk to and reassure him all the time. An anxious new parent may forget the talking part and just concentrate on the technique. Yet the reassuring sound of your voice may be more important than the deftness of your handling. A baby who obviously dislikes bright light should be kept in a dimly lit room, and the light only gradually increased to the level at which she is happy with it. Even those who have had very straightforward deliveries may screw up their eyes in light, while others do not seem to object.

When our twins were born (at home) my husband immediately noticed that Tess disliked the light, so when she was not in bed with me she spent her time in a crib half inside my wardrobe. Nell did not object in the same way and the ordinary lighting of the bedroom seemed fine for her.

When they went outside in the garden, a couple of days later, they were in a cot with hanging draperies and under the spreading boughs of an apple tree so that we could control the light till it was right for them both to be able to open their eyes comfortably when they were in their alert state, and look around and explore.

If you have ever seen a baby who is allowed to cry for long periods before being picked up and fed you can guess at the sheer animal terror and pain she is going through. I think we underestimate what a newborn baby may be enduring when pangs of hunger are not satisfied. A baby who has had a difficult birth should never have to wait to be fed, until she is old enough to understand that food and loving arms are coming soon and can use crying as a deliberate message to which she knows there will be an appropriate response.

THE SLEEPY BABY

A drowsy baby may have had a difficult birth because she was subjected to analgesic or anaesthetic drugs which reached her through the mother's blood stream. All pain-relieving drugs taken by the mother pass through the placenta to the baby, although some in proportions much lower than in the mother's own blood. One of the worst offenders is pethidine (Demerol in the USA) a narcotic drug which dopes both mother and baby. The mother may come round from it fairly quickly after delivery, but the baby's immature liver does not excrete it so easily. This may mean that the baby is un-responsive and sleepy for the first few days after delivery, just when the mother is trying to establish breastfeeding, and sucking patterns may be affected for at least ten days.[3] Babies who have received one dose of sedation during labour suck more slowly and weakly and get less milk than those whose mothers have not been sedated.[4] When a mother has received analgesic drugs in labour she is more likely to develop en-gorged breasts afterwards because her baby tends not to suckle vigorously.[5] Pethidine is the most widely used obstet-ric drug in Britain, and this can be a major problem for mothers.

Hospitals are very hot places, especially postnatal wards, because paediatricians are concerned to prevent heat loss in newborns. A baby has a good deal of surface area in relation to its size, and heat loss occurs all over this surface. A baby also has a very large head in relation to the rest of its body, and heat loss takes place particularly over the surface of the head, which is often uncovered. This is why your baby may come to you dressed up in an extraordinary ugly bonnet or head covering, or even wrapped in bacon foil. If she spends part of her time in a nursery, this may be hotter still. The result may be that it is very difficult to wake the baby up at all. A little judicious stimulation accompanied by slight cooling down is then called for. Unwrap the baby, talk to her, stroke and massage her, play little games, get her feet out in the open and let her feel some counterpressure against them. This last trick helps especially. Get into a face-to-face position so that when at last she does open her eyes she sees her fascinating mother. When eventually she starts to suck do not expect a long feed. Little and often is the best guide. A drowsy baby cannot keep up the sustained effort to take a full feed, and it is better to think in terms of a number of small temptations to the appetite, like a Chinese feast. Premature and juandiced babies are usually rather sleepy and unresponsive.

When a baby is sleepy the mother may find it difficult to cope with her own feelings at not being able to give her baby anything she really wants or which excites him. It is not very rewarding for her when she turns to talk to someone, for example, to find that the baby has slipped off her breast and does not seek it again. The mother of a sleepy baby needs a good deal of emotional support.

THE JAUNDICED BABY

About half of all babies develop jaundice which reaches a peak on about the third to fifth day of life. This is nearly always *physiologic jaundice* which occurs when the red blood cells which the baby needed for development in the uterus with its reduced oxygen supply are broken down as the baby's

metabolism becomes adapted to life outside the uterus. Bilirubin, or bile pigment, which is yellow in colour, cannot be
excreted efficiently by the newborn's immature liver and
colours the skin so that the baby looks suntanned. A premature or low-birth-weight baby may be even less able than the
full-term baby to handle the bilirubin, so jaundice may be
more marked.

The jaundiced baby readily becomes dehydrated, so should
be given constant small feeds, small because she is also sleepy
and is unlikely to keep awake for long and may fall asleep
shortly after beginning to suckle. If the baby is very drowsy
she may need waking every two or three hours to suckle.
When the bilirubin count is high feeding difficulties often
start at this time, as one needs great patience to cope with a
drowsy, 'floppy' baby, and the mother's anxiety may be great.
If you need to wake the baby, freshen her up with a wash and
change which will provide a stimulus for her to suckle.

The paediatrician may decide to treat the jaundice with
phototherapy and the baby is placed naked under a fluores-
cent light, usually with the eyes bandaged to protect them. If
sunlight is available this is an excellent treatment for jaundice. Unfortunately many hospital nurseries are designed so
that babies cannot be put in the sunlight, and in some there
are no windows to the outside at all.

Pregnanediol jaundice, sometimes incorrectly called 'breast
milk jaundice' starts later and reaches a peak at ten to thir-
teen days. This is discussed on page 152.

If your baby is having light treatment, remove the eye
covering before you breastfeed as eye contact between
mother and baby is important. Talk to her and give her a
good deal of loving touch to try to compensate for the sensory deprivation which results from having the eyes covered.

THE PREMATURE OR LOW-BIRTH-WEIGHT BABY
(See also 'The baby gets ill', page 139.)

This baby may not suckle at first because the birth was
tiring and rest is the first need. One who weighs less
than about 2 lb will not have a suckling reflex, but babies

who weigh over 3½ lb sometimes produce a strong sucking reflex. Babies obviously vary in the extent to which they suck while they are still in the uterus and some are born ready to carry on doing what they have already been enjoying in the uterus.

Some premature babies are not able to suckle or become exhausted if they do so for more than a few minutes. The paediatrician may decide on tube feeding until the reflex is established so that the baby does not become worn out. A fine tube is passed through the baby's nose and down into the stomach and is left in place. The baby who is being tube-fed can be fed on breast milk if the mother expresses her milk with a breast pump starting the day following delivery. Many large hospitals now have milk banks where donor breast milk is stored to be used for babies in special need of it. Expression with a breast pump will stimulate the mother's milk supply so that she is ready to take over whenever she can if her baby starts with breast milk from the bank. The baby can be given breast milk by tube and can then have a bottle or go straight to the breast.

When a baby is very premature and the chances are that it will not live, it is up to the mother to decide whether she feels able to commit herself to sending milk to the nursery in this way or whether the experience will prove too painful for her should the baby die. Some women have found that it helped them to do everything they could for their babies, and enabled them to cope with the deep feelings of guilt which a mother experiences when her baby is premature. The questions always in her mind are, 'Could I have done anything to prevent my baby being premature? Did anything I did cause her to be premature?' and if the baby dies, 'Is there anything else I could have done so that my baby would have survived?' To give your milk to a baby, even if it does live only a short while, is a positive act which can be entered on and also allows the parents to see the baby as a real being to be mourned. Grieving is most difficult and painful when there is no real being to mourn.

Since babies quickly grow to prefer the super-stimulus of a bottle teat to the mother's nipple there is an advantage in introducing short and frequent breastfeeds for the premature baby as soon as possible.

Premature babies need stimulating. Marshall Klaus and John Kennell, paediatricians who have drawn attention to the impact of early separation between a baby and its parents on the later development of the family, say that if a premature baby is fondled, rocked or cuddled daily during its stay in the nursery 'he has fewer apneoic periods, increased weight gain, a smaller number of stools, as well as an advance in some areas of higher central nervous system functioning, which persists for many months after discharge.'[6]

Although they tend to be drowsy, premature babies often startle easily and demonstrate a reflex response (the Moro reflex) in which they fling their arms up as if they are afraid that you are about to drop them. This can be very worrying for the mother who thinks she must be handling her baby wrongly and it can soon sap her confidence.

Even the baby who must remain in an incubator can be touched and stroked. Not only do all babies need cuddling, but their mothers and fathers need to hold them to get to know and *feel* that they are mothers and fathers. Body contact and close flesh-to-flesh contact of bare skin is especially important in helping both mother and baby enjoy times at the breast. Not all hospitals see this as important, and nurses are sometimes concerned that the mother may get anxious if she attempts to feed and is not successful, or think the feeding 'challenge' is best left till the baby is approaching normal weight. Yet the baby who is in special care particularly needs this kind of loving and should not be deprived of it even if it has to take place in short periods when the baby can be taken out of an incubator. A woman can do a great deal by her own calm attitude and obvious sense of pleasure in the baby to reassure nurses that she can cope and avoid making them anxious that she is tiring the baby with what they may see as the demands she is making on him. Ask if you can help with your baby's care, even if it is only to steady a piece of apparatus while the nurse does something. You may like to pour the milk into the feeding tube for the baby. As you get to know staff better and are a familiar figure around the nursery you will probably be able to do a number of things to help your baby.

Yet it is difficult to feel that a baby really belongs to you when it is covered with tubes and wires, or even to *want* to pick it up and hold it close if it is scrawny and pathetic. Or the mother and father may be so appalled at what one man described as 'the horrible tubes' that they 'want to wrench the bloody things off'. 'I watched the birth', his wife added, 'and when they discovered she was ill it was very difficult to hand over to doctors and nurses.' The parents can help each other by discussing their real feelings together and not trying to simulate emotions they do not feel or to disguise the negative ones they may be experiencing. Painful as it is, it may be an important occasion for growth in their relationship.

It is sometimes hard to face up to a situation which you realize is far from ideal, a baby who is bucketed into life at a disadvantage, who looks different from other babies and, because there are so many experts around, is apparently not the parents' responsibility at all.

It is understandable that some mothers and fathers feel they have to escape this, leave the professionals to cope and even to try and forget the baby exists. Since some hospitals are organized so it is the father who can visit the special care baby unit more regularly than the mother, and she is left more or less stranded on a different floor of the building, he may find it easier to relate to the baby at first than she does. When a premature baby is discharged from hospital the trauma has been so great for some mothers that they do not want their babies and refuse to take them home.

When a baby has been very premature it is also difficult to believe that it ever will be all right and a mother may see her normal, thriving baby as in some way 'deformed'.[7] Some women are over-protective about children who were premature many years after they need special cherishing. Some see them as under-achieving and 'backward', and probably actually make them 'difficult' because of this attitude. Battered babies are very likely to have been premature, but extended contact between the mother and her premature baby from the earliest days, even if she can only touch him through the armholes in an incubator at first, helps her to have much more positive feelings and to care for her child in a way which is satisfying for both.[8]

THE BABY WHO STARTLES EASILY

Your baby will let you know the kind of care and the type of environment she needs. Some babies seem to want a great deal of life going on around them from the beginning. Others are not ready for a full social life and the noise and bustle of a family or admiring visitors. Follow your baby's lead, respect her individuality and you can work out together the right setting for feeds.

A baby delivered after the mother has had an epidural may startle in this way. The baby who startles readily, jerks, trembles, turns pale and cries, benefits from firm holding and slow movements, and a constantly warm atmosphere, and may be much happier when swaddled or bound in a flannelette sheet or blanket. Lift her for a feed *before* she has begun to cry whenever possible, since feelings of hunger and her own crying may make her over-react, and keep her wrapped until about to change her. There is no need to make everyone be quiet in the vicinity, and a low background hum or buzz of conversation and activity is more peaceful for your baby than complete silence interrupted by sudden, intrusive noises. If a bath is upsetting for her, keep bathing till she is a few weeks older.

As the baby's nervous system matures she will be able to cope with more casual handling and greater stimulus.

TWINS

Because twins provide double the stimulus to the breasts they are often easy to breastfeed and the mother of twins finds that she has lashings of milk. She also often discovers that she has an enormous appetite and thirst but does not put on weight.

The babies can be fed at the same time or separately.

When fed together it is usually easiest to tuck their legs under your arms, with their heads side by side on a pillow on your lap.

If they are fed separately, however, they each get the same amount of individual attention. They are different people with different needs and may have different rhythms of suckling. Each of the twins may correspond to any of the types of babies described in this chapter and they should be observed and treated as individuals. It is also less of a juggling act to feed them separately as, if one is finished before the other and needs to be sat up or put over your shoulder to deal with air bubbles, the only way of doing it is to toss her like a pancake.

Twins are probably more likely than single babies to go short of comfort sucking. A good milk supply and a ready letdown reflex provides nutrition, but the strong rate of flow of the milk and the fact that the mother is very busy with two babies curtails time at the breast for non-nutritive sucking. There is a case for offering a dummy if it seems that a twin needs to suck more, but avoid leaving a baby plugged with a dummy for long periods of time. Babies are human beings and need human beings with them, not rubber and plastic artefacts.

Books often advise the mother of twins to have pieces of ribbon of different colours or other means of identification attached to safety pins to fix to the bra strap so that each baby is started on a different side at each feed. It sounds a good idea until one actually has to remember to do it and to change them over even though the door bell and the telephone are ringing together. There is no need to give the babies different sides at every feed.

Although you may be advised to breastfeed one baby and bottle feed the other, or to do so alternately, avoid this if you possibly can as it makes for much more work unless you have constant help with the babies. The most important thing to remember, even though you may be very tired at times, especially if you have older children as well, is that the more often the babies feed, *the more milk will be produced*. A mother cannot 'save' her milk by missing a feed. The only place breast milk can be stored is in the fridge. One woman wrote to me that although she had breastfed four babies rather unsatisfactorily before, she did not learn this until her twins, numbers five and six, came along! If you need to increase your milk supply in order to feed one the best way of doing so is to suckle both as often as possible. My twenty-four hour peak production plan (page 132) usually works in twelve hours with twins.

It helps to be in touch with another mother of twins, and your general practitioner, the staff at the hospital or your local National Childbirth Trust teacher may be able to let you have the names and phone numbers of other women who have breastfed twins with whom you can share experiences.

THE BABY WHO FIGHTS THE BREAST

I doubt whether any babies are innately 'aggressive' and it is important to avoid labelling your baby as being 'angry' or 'hostile', as 'like her father', or as having any other special character which will affect how you interact with and interpret her needs, perhaps for ever after.

A baby who struggles at the breast may do so for several reasons. One thing that may be happening is that she may be finding it *difficult to breathe*. Some babies are still stopped up with mucus in the first couple of days and need further suctioning or draining with their heads lower than their bottoms. Sneezing is the spontaneous way in which they clear this mucus.

If you are engorged or have large breasts breast tissue may be in the way of the baby's nostrils. Although you need have no fear that your baby can suffocate (she will just turn her head away if she is uncomfortable) it can help her to feed more easily if the mother sees that her nose is clear of the breast by dimpling the breast with one or two fingers, and that the baby is propped up so that her own upper lip is not occluding her nostrils. With a tiny baby this is simple to do if she is placed on a pillow on the mother's lap. Neither the mother nor a helper should hold the baby's head. Simply support it in the crook of the arm, unless you prefer the position described on page 58, in which case the hand *cradles* the head but does not hold it.

Or the baby may be *'jumpy' and excitable*, sometimes because she has had a difficult birth or is insufficiently mature to cope with all the intense stimuli of life outside the uterus. (See also 'The baby who startles', page 83.)

If your baby is easily overstimulated try gently rousing her for feeds before she is actively searching for food, and put her straight to the breast without unwrapping her, in a peaceful, quiet atmosphere. Dim lights or a shaded window and soft music may help you both.

Sometimes the let-down reflex is extremely powerful and *the milk comes very fast* and suddenly and pours into a baby who is sucking strongly, who then chokes, draws back, screams and fights the breast. See page 123.

It can help to give the vigorous, excitable baby a little boiled, cooled water or warm, weak, strained tea made with fresh washed mint, and for the mother to press on her breast so that the first rush of milk is expressed, until her baby has learned that it works better when she suckles more gently. Half a minute's sucking time with mint tea on a few occasions will probably relax both mother and baby ready for the real feed. If the baby anticipates a breastfeed when held in her mother's arms, she can hold her facing outward on her lap for this drink from a bottle to avoid confusion.

But a baby may start suckling and then draw away in agitation because although milk is present in the breast and the mother can feel her breast firm and full of milk, little or none is being conveyed to the baby. If this happens to you check first that your baby is really 'fixed' on the nipple and areola. See page 54.

Stasis of milk can occur when a mother is feeding with her arms pressed against her sides splinting her breast with her arms, and can also contribute to difficulty in the baby getting the milk. Often just a small part of the breast is made available to the baby, who seems to be getting milk from only part of it. Undo the bra flap completely or take off the bra and try a more luxurious, spread-out position. Uncover the baby's hands so that she can touch and explore your breast.

Often this mother, worried that she has insufficient milk, is having rest in bed and is making minimal arm movements. She needs the rest, but she also needs to make energetic arm movements; with modern labour-saving devices we get less and less exercise in our everyday lives. Vigorous walking with arms swinging, the baby nestled in a carrier against your body, is good. Although it is important to avoid getting exhausted, exercise till you get a glow, with free movement of the arms. There is more about stasis on page 117.

THE HANDICAPPED BABY

It is physically difficult for a baby with hare lip and cleft palate to suckle, although this depends very much on the degree of cleft palate. Some babies can *learn* to suckle successfully although it is difficult at first. The mother may find that a soft latex nipple shield allows the baby to get a good mouthful. The Natural Nursing Nipple Shield can be effective, and is obtainable from the National Childbirth Trust.[9]

Some surgeons repair the cleft palate within a few days of birth. Others do so after about three months. Early surgery results in a baby which the mother may find it easier to feed both because she looks normal and how babies *should* be, and because the baby can suck easily. Following surgery the mother needs to express her milk with a breast pump. If she is still in hospital or has gone into hospital to be with her baby an electric pump should be available.

Many babies who have Down's syndrome are very difficult to feed because they are so sleepy, and any mentally handicapped baby may need to be wakened for feeds every three or four hours and then coaxed to suckle. This drowsiness should not be confused with that characteristic of many newborn babies when their mothers have received analgesic drugs in labour, a condition which is alleviated after a few days.

THE BABY WHO REFUSES TO SUCKLE
AT ONE BREAST

Sometimes a baby prefers one breast to the other and makes this clear by avoiding suckling at the other. If the mother is right handed this is often her right breast. It seems that she can position the baby more easily using her right hand to help her than her left. It may help to start suckling on the less liked side first. The trick which allows the mother to slip her baby on to the 'difficult' side is to place him with his face towards the breast and his body and legs slid under her arm on the same side.

The draught of milk may not be equally strong in both breasts, so that the baby may have to work harder at one side and becomes impatient before the milk comes in. Talking or singing to her while you wait for the flow to become established may help. A hot face flannel rested over the breast immediately before putting the baby to that side may help trigger the reflex.

THE BABY WHO NEVER WANTS TO
STOP SUCKLING

Probably more babies are like this than their mothers ever care to admit. It speaks well for the experience of being at the breast that many babies enjoy it so much that they do not want to do anything else, and as soon as you make a slight movement to detach them, even though they are apparently fast asleep, they snap their mouths open and on to the breast again as if they were desperately hungry.

The mother, especially if it is her first baby, quickly feels that he may be really undernourished, and that she cannot be providing enough milk. It only needs someone well-meaning to ask, 'Are you sure you have sufficient milk?' or 'Is that baby having enough?' for her confidence to be completely shattered.

She needs to distinguish between *nutritional* and *comfort suckling. Babies need both.* When a baby is enjoying comfort suckling she often merely nibbles the nipple or puts on a pretty good performance of nutritional suckling but without any jaw movement. If you look carefully you will see that she is not swallowing. Or she may get the knack of pushing the nipple a little away with the front part of her tongue so that there is reduced pressure on the areola and hence over the milk pools and she can suck without drinking. Some babies do this even when they want to feed because they have been fed from bottles with large holes in the teat and have learned to control the flow of milk in this manner.

Once the mother begins to observe the signs of comfort suckling she will develop the confidence to know when her baby is full up and when if she wants to put him down she can do so, even though he may grumble a bit. Sucking a dummy or his fingers may soothe a baby who wants more comfort suckling or close holding, but it will not quieten one who is hungry. A baby who is not hungry may also be contented when carried against the mother's or father's body in a baby carrier and may be prepared to forgo constant suckling as long as he is with you like this. One advantage of baby carriers is that if the mother positions a baby correctly in it against her breast she can let him suckle even while she is carrying on doing other things.

When putting down a baby who is like this do so with a firm, slow, rhythmic movement and avoid dithering. Wrap her up and if she starts to grizzle, rock the cradle or pat her bottom firmly with steady, definite movements and the rhythm of the ticking of a grandfather clock. See also Chapter 9, page 95.

THE VOMITING BABY

Fortunately a breastfed baby's regurgitation smells all right. That from an artificially fed baby smells sour. All babies vomit sometimes, often when they have been gulping the feed. Some babies vomit often and seem to thrive on it. But when a breastfed baby vomits this is usually simple 'possetting', a delightful word to describe a messy thing; one can think of it more as 'spilling over'. Pressure on a baby's tummy following a feed can lead to some being brought back. If a baby has possetted she may have a space which needs to be filled again and will want to suckle a little longer.

Projectile vomiting is rare. There is no doubt about it at all if your baby is vomiting like this, because the milk shoots back as if fired from a gun. Let a paediatrician see the baby immediately. Some babies have projectile vomiting but are physically perfect. They only vomit in this way after going a long time between feeds, and the mother may be able to avoid it by not letting her baby get so frantically hungry. If the baby is getting bigger and plumping out and is producing wet nappies there is nothing organically wrong. Treat the baby like the one who is excitable, described on page 86. Take it for granted that your milk comes fast and try expression and mint tea.

THE BABY WITH THRUSH

Breastfed babies are less likely than artificially fed babies to get thrush in their mouths, because the yeast which causes the growth of this fungus is inhibited by acetic and lactic acids in human milk. But a baby can pick up thrush during its passage down the birth canal from the mother's vagina and in turn infect her nipples, which become sore. Thrush is similar to athlete's foot, and looks like scraps of curdled milk in the baby's mouth and on her gums and tongue. When one is gently scraped it bleeds. It makes feeding painful for the baby. This is not to be confused with tiny white marks called 'epithelial pearls' which may also be in the baby's mouth. Thrush can also cause nappy rash.

Let your doctor see the baby. Treat the nipples by submerging each in a solution of bicarbonate of soda: one teaspoonful in a cup of cooled, boiled water after feeds. Also see the section on sore nipples on page 111.

THE BABY WHO BITES

There comes a time when the baby discovers she can bite the nipple and produce a surprising response from the mother. An intelligent baby is, above all, experimental, and this proves interesting and great fun. Everything about the mother changes in a second, the expression on her face, the way she is holding the baby, her breathing, and she may even cry out. Of course, the baby wants to do it again to see if the same results can be produced.

People sometimes ask a breastfeeding mother, 'What will you do when she has teeth? Won't she bite you?' But babies can bite perfectly well on the sensitive tissue on the nipple without having any teeth, and it is usually before they come through that this developmental stage is reached.

The impulse to bite is a normal part of growing, but the mother has to know how to handle the situation. I have read in some books on child-rearing that she should promptly strike her baby, so making it clear that this is not allowed. But it is completely unnecessary for her to over-react in such a retaliatory, vindictive way. She has only to draw back a bit and say firmly and quietly 'No'. She can draw away because the baby almost invariably on seeing the initial startled re-action lets go of the nipple and may be smiling up at her. The baby will already have received a signal from her physical re-sponse, the way she automatically grips her as well as with-drawing, but it is a good idea to link this with words spoken firmly. This definite 'no' is one of the messages that the grow-ing baby will have to understand in other situations too.

A baby who needs to bite can be given other things to bite – a teething ring or a hard-baked crust (not raw carrots, which can cause choking).

This is not the time to wean. Much is happening in the relationship between mother and baby at this stage that has to be lived through. It is important, too, that the baby learns that the mother *goes on being the same kind of person* and cannot be destroyed. I am not referring to the real death of the mother here, but to her changing and in some way reject-ing the child, becoming a withdrawn relatively uninvolved mother whereas previously she was a loving, caring one, for example. Power is frightening to wield. As the small child discovers power she needs to know from experience that the world does not collapse round her, and that even though she does things that are disapproved or 'naughty', disaster does not strike. All human beings have to learn how to cope with their own aggressive impulses and not to be shattered by them.

Aggression is not just a power which is unleashed towards an enemy; it is one which can take over the person experiencing it too, and can be a terrifying force which threatens self-destruction. Because the mother continues as the same kind of mother and can survive the baby's fantasy destruction of her, she is able to help the baby cope with aggression and to start living in a world on which the growing child can act decisively without fear of destroying everything around her or of being herself consumed in the holocaust. This is an important part of psychological maturation that continues through to adulthood.

A baby is not just a cuddly bundle, nor an animal with primitive, compelling instincts (although sometimes it may seem like that), nor only the passive *object* of parental care and concern; nor a doll to be dressed up and put down when the parents are tired of playing with it; nor a pet to be trained and rewarded for good behaviour and fitted conveniently into their lives. It is not a gift which can be returned to the shop, discreetly forgotten or exchanged for another, not just Johnny's brother or Peggy's youngest or Mary's grand-daughter; a baby is not a glue which can ensure that a marriage continues, a certificate of potency or womanliness, or a projection of the parents' personalities who can, through their child, be the people they never were and achieve the things they never succeeded in doing in their own lives. The baby is its own self.

A baby is unique right from the start. The mother's and father's first task and their continuing responsibility is to get to know their baby as a person.

9. Sleeping, waking and crying

Babies sleep as much as they need to. Sometimes parents worry that their babies are not getting enough sleep. What they are usually saying is that *they* do not get enough respite from the baby's demands, or have enough sleep themselves. This is a quite reasonable complaint about the upheaval that this often delightful stranger has caused in their lives. But so far as the baby is concerned they should understand that she will sleep when and for as long as she needs.

This is one of the extraordinary things about babies, that they can drop off when they are ready in however an apparently uncomfortable position they are lying or sitting and whatever the rumpus going on around them. Similarly, they wake up when they are ready even though everyone in the house is going round on tip-toe and 'shushing' each other.

But it is difficult not to become anxious when a baby spends long hours crying or fussing. It seems so exhausting for the baby, and yet she does not sleep, or dozes for a few minutes and then comes to and starts crying again. This often happens in the evening and may be called 'three-month colic' because this behaviour tends to disappear at about three months. There is no evidence that most of these 'colicky' babies are in any pain. *All* babies draw up their knees when they cry. It does not mean that they have a tummy-ache. But it is clear that they are irritable. Parents rack their brains to think what they can do with these babies and try one activity after another. Maybe they are doing just what is required; the baby is asking for a great deal and varied kinds of stimulus and they are kept busy offering new kinds. Looked at in this way, this is an important learning period for the baby. The odd thing too, is that these babies thrive and do not appear to suffer from any lack of sleep, although if these wakeful periods extend into the night and the early hours of the morning, their parents do.

Most new babies cry when they wake. This does not mean that they are unhappy in the sense that we experience unhappiness. They are providing an imperative signal to their caretakers that there is an urgent need to satisfy hunger. The cry has an important function in the survival of the human species. Without it a new mother might forget she had a baby or might not be aware of when she should feed it. But it can be distressing to parents to hear their newborn sounding so miserable. Here again, there is a biological function, and their distress makes them want to do something about it, so they stop whatever they are doing and take care of the baby.

Later on the baby lies for minutes without crying, just gazing around the room and at the interesting things which have been hung around her cot. But by then the parents have usually learned their caretaking roles well and know that when the baby cries she needs attention. They have come through this initial learning period and patterns of parenting have been established.

Some couples believe that if they are being good parents the baby should never cry. They may have been influenced by the ideas of Frederick Leboyer[1] and feel that even at birth a baby 'should' not cry, but smile. Leboyer, however, says that it is *prolonged* crying which seems to him wrong, and that if the baby is cared for lovingly and with consideration and gentleness the baby becomes contented. Some babies cry more energetically than others anyway, because they are different people. A mentally handicapped baby may hardly ever cry, and when she does it is only a soft reed-like warble. (Other mentally handicapped babies *do* cry, but in an abnormal shrill scream.) I remember two mothers who were feeling frantic about their newborn babies' energetic crying meeting again a woman who had been in their antenatal class who had given birth to a sweet little baby suffering from Down's syndrome (mongolism), who never cried. The handicapped baby would have been some people's ideal of a 'good' baby if she had not been handicapped. Afterwards, the women who had normal crying babies said they felt so relieved and were better prepared to cope with the babies they had.

Books sometimes tell their readers how long babies should sleep. Unfortunately the babies have never read these books. Studies of babies' sleeping have revealed that in fact they sleep far less than used to be thought. Averages can be misleading, but one research project showed that a newborn baby sleeps sixteen hours twenty minutes out of the twenty-four in the first week after birth, and in the sixteenth week is down to under fifteen hours.[2] This means that even the newborn baby is awake for about a third of the time, and some sleep far less than this.

No one can force a baby to sleep. All that can be done is to create the conditions in which it is easiest for her to sleep. One way is to have a background of *rhythmic sound*, which, perhaps because it is closer to the conditions the baby experienced inside the uterus, may be more soporific in effect than complete silence. Any household machine, music or even a regular background of human conversation can do this. Perhaps this is the origin of the lullaby, which uses the comforting effect of the frequencies of the human voice combined with the rhythms of musical cadence. You can make and adapt your own lullabies, and it does not matter if they are nonsense.

If you have no music available, or feel the need to be quiet yourself and take a bath or read a book, anything that whirrs or hums is likely to interest the baby, a dishwasher or washing machine, or dryer or vacuum cleaner. If a washer or dryer does not reverberate too much you can even put the baby in a carry cot or basket right on the machine, but be sure the machine is not steamy or too hot.

Babies tend to sleep or, if they are in an alert period, their crying stops when they hear a regular sound similar to the beat of the human heart, that is about sixty to eighty beats a minute. Dr Hajime Murooka's record (Sleep Softly in the Womb, EMI) of a mother's aorta and other intra-uterine sounds also has an almost magical effect on babies, and can send a whole nursery of newborns gently to sleep.

When a new mother is going through a difficult period of extreme anxiety or depression associated with her relationship with the baby (which almost invariably means that the baby finds it difficult to drop off to sleep and stay asleep) I sometimes tuck the mother up in bed for a good sleep while I rest the baby beside me on my own bed and get on with typing an article or book. Typing itself produces the kind of regular sound that babies seem to like. If the baby is crying I play Dr Murooka's record as I work, and without fail a baby under six weeks of age quietens and either lies listening or goes to sleep. After that age the sounds are less effective, but still work sometimes. Anybody can do this and it is an easy way of soothing a baby.

Rocking, which presumably produces an effect similar to that obtained *in utero* when the baby is rocked in the maternal pelvis, can also be effective at sending a baby off to sleep. In antique shops you can still find old rocking cradles with a piece attached so that the mother could rock it with her foot while doing other work with her hands. Victorian cradles were often adapted from the coffers in which young girls stored the linen and nightwear ready for marriage. They were dual function objects, rather like the patchwork marriage bedspread filled with cut-up love letters! It would be a good thing to make a modern version of the rocking cradle. The up-and-down movement is best if it is only about three inches. If a woman rests her fingers on the edge of the big bones which form that part of her pelvis which is above her outer thighs, and then rocks the pelvic cradle forward and back, alternately tightening and releasing abdominal and buttock muscles, she will discover that this bone moves up and down by approximately three inches as she does so. So this is what the baby was used to when inside her uterus.

Rocking chairs are comforting both for the parent who is hoping a child will go to sleep and for the baby. These are not difficult to buy, whether old or modern, but if you want to use it for breastfeeding it is easier for you if the arm rests are low. When they are high the baby's head may be banged against one inadvertently, and it is tricky to position your arms so that they are comfortable with the baby at the breast. In a study of rocking it was discovered that babies like best to be rocked at about sixty beats a minute, again in a rhythm similar to the human heartbeat.[3] But you do not have to clock-watch while rocking. The right rhythm is the one you find works for you and your baby.

As they are learning to organize their behaviour babies appreciate corresponding patterns in their environment. This seems to help them create their own sequences of behaviour in terms of waking, sleeping, feeding and so on. It is useless to try and impose patterns on babies, but by introducing *patterns of caretaking behaviour* which are repeated over and over again in the same manner, babies come to anticipate their mothers' actions. After the first few weeks of life the baby knows the sequence of action by her mother which leads to suckling at the breast, and may make anticipatory movements. In much the same way a regular sequence of actions before sleep-time prepares the baby to anticipate sleep.

This may be one reason why if many different people are constantly caring for a baby, each one doing things in a different way, development is often retarded.[4] This does not matter in a traditional society, where grandmother, aunt, older sister, and the other relatives all do much the same thing as the mother, because there are culturally patterned ways of caring for babies which are so powerful that people do not even need to think what they are doing for the most part. In our own society some of the deprivation from which babies suffer when they do not have the constant attention of one caretaker, which has been attributed to an emotional reaction to loss of the mother,[5] may be due to never being able to experience continuity in the way they are handled, soothed, fed, changed, and so on. As a mother learns to care for a baby she develops specific patterns of behaviour to such an extent that she may correct her husband who only occasionally looks after the baby when he holds or puts him down in a way that is subtly different from hers, and against which the baby protests. When two people, mother and father, both share more or less equally in caring for a baby, he quickly adapts to two distinctive patterns.

Patterns of caretaking can be deliberately created to help the baby sleep at appropriate times. The parents introduce ritual before sleeping, and this ritual becomes anticipated

by the baby. All ritual is symbolic, has meaning beyond the
meaning of its different constituent actions, and in effect says
something in an often non-verbal language. *Ritualized patterns* of parental behaviour as the baby is put down to sleep
are saying 'Time to sleep now' and introduce the assurance of
security which comes from well-known, often repeated caretaking actions.

One action of this kind might be to *wrap the baby firmly*.
She comes to associate this with sleep. Traditionally European babies were swaddled. With our modern emphasis on
freedom and self-expression this has gone out of fashion. But
many babies seem to like being securely wrapped in a flan-
elette sheet or shawl and sleep better when this is done.[6] If
parents keep this for times when it is particularly desirable
that the baby sleeps, and do not do it when it does not much
matter, it is likely to be more effective.

Babies quickly come to associate *darkness* or the light being dimmed with sleep-time too. At first they make no distinction between night and day, but by two to three weeks a
baby may develop diurnal rhythms, sleeping longer at night
than in the day. It is as if the biological clock is automatically
adjusted to fit in with the social enviroment. The baby is
taking one of the first big steps in acculturation. Some babies
take much longer to adapt to the culture, but generally, if the
parents give firm and unconfused messages, will soon start
to sleep longer between feeds at night until at last at four or
five months old (sometimes earlier, sometimes later) she
sleeps through the night.

Unless the parents want to institute a night feed as play-
time, it is sensible to give muted *low-key attention at night*,
reducing stimuli passing between the parents and the baby,
keeping light low, sounds unexciting, and having everything
at hand so that the baby (and the parents) can settle off again
as quickly as possible.

Conveying to the baby that now is sleep-time is also easier
if she is *put down in a special position* when you would like
her to sleep. If the baby is put down on her front only when it
is intended that she shall sleep she associates this position
with the cessation of social activities for the time being. She

may not like it sometimes, and may protest, but she knows what you mean.

Whatever ritual patterns the parents decide to link with giving the message that it is now sleep-time, it is essential to start on activities which can be kept up, and which are not suddenly omitted because a special nightlight, musical box or sleeping place is no longer available. It is important to consider how you will cope when you are staying in someone else's home or a hotel, or camping.

There is a marked cultural contrast between Western industrialized societies where babies are supposed to lie sleeping in prams or cots, and peasant societies and those of the Third World where babies are carried round close to the mother's body, and later often by older siblings, and are an integral part of all activity that is going on.[7] The African or Indian mother with her baby bound to her body by a strip of cloth works with her baby being tipped forward as she bends, swaying with her body movements, jogging up and down as she pounds millet or coffee beans, and being suckled whenever he seems to need feeding. These babies hardly ever cry. This can be explained in several ways, but predominant among them is the constant rhythmic stimulation provided by the work environment, the close physical connection between mother and baby, and the satisfaction of hunger and thirst as soon as the need arises.

As life-styles change in the West more and more mothers are adopting something of these child-care practices, and find that it fits in well with their own way of life. Whenever I lecture in the USA I am struck by the number of babies carried in slings nestled beneath their mothers' breasts who sleep and suckle without making any disturbance, while their mothers participate fully in the workshops.

For the breastfeeding mother a baby carrier allows her arms to be free to continue daily activities in and outside her home and gives the baby the comfort of her continuous physical presence. The mother need never worry about whether the baby is awake or asleep and whether or not he needs her, because she is right there. And the baby has a valuable opportunity when in an alert state to learn about the extraordinary world in which he is already playing an active part, not segregated to the nursery or at the end of the garden cut off from the excitement in a pram, but in the hub of it all.

There are many different kinds of carriers on the market now. But choose one which supports the new baby's head and which grows with the baby, as they continue to be useful at the toddler stage, especially if you go for long walks or to outdoor activities at which a small child gets bored or tired.

The National Childbirth Trust[8] recommends a carrier called Easy Rider, which can be used from the time the baby is born until she is about two years old, and worn on the front or back. The American Snugli is a more sophisticated and luxurious, and also much more expensive, model, available in beautifully coloured corduroys. This is available from Sarah Campbell, 20 Ashchurch Terrace, London W 12 (tel. 01 743 8374).

With baby carriers both parents have a mobility which it is impossible to have while coping with a huge pram or even a carrycot with wheels, though these can be very useful in the car.

Sleep does not all take place at the same level. Most newborn babies sleep deeply for only about twenty or twenty-five minutes at a time, and then this is replaced by sleep in which they make many little movements, twitch, breathe at different rates, blink and look as if they are responding to intense inner states or perhaps dreams. This is REM sleep, that is, sleep during which there are rapid eye movements. When adults are deprived of REM sleep by being woken up as soon as their eyelids start fluttering or their eyes move they become very exhausted. Babies, too, seem to need this sleep. Rudolph Schaffer suggests that this increase in nerve cell activity, and the blood flow in the brain which accompanies it,

may be essential for the normal growth of brain tissue. The foetus, shielded by the womb, and the young baby, still relatively helpless, get little or no environmental stimulation; REM sleep may serve as a built-in self-stimulation system that periodically provides activity and so helps prepare the brain for dealing with 'real' stimulation. Once this real stimulation is provided ... REM sleep is no longer so vital. Maternal stimulation has come to take over from REM-type stimulation.[9]

The breastfeeding mother who is watching for her baby to wake up should not misinterpret the signs of REM sleep as indicating that the baby is waking and should be picked up. A mother who is trying to increase her milk supply by feeding frequently can become discouraged if she lifts up her baby at the first moment she stirs and then discovers that she is not ready to suck and refuses the breast. If you do this, let the baby drift off again, continuing to hold her close or to stay near, and after some minutes she will probably wake properly. Do not, whatever you do, attempt to joggle the baby awake or slap her feet as some nurses do.

New babies often find the journey down into sleep difficult, and may jerk and cry out as they are beginning to slip into sleep. An anxious mother rushes to pick her baby up when she does this, wondering if a safety pin is sticking in her, or she is too hot or too cold, or has 'wind'. But if the baby tends to do this as part of the complicated process of going to sleep and the mother continues to rouse her every time it happens, both of them eventually become worn out and frustrated.

Some babies regularly cry for ten or fifteen minutes after the parent thinks they have been settled, and continue this for some minutes. It is important to observe and discover your baby's behaviour. Sometimes when there are sleeping problems an anxious parent is not *letting* a baby get to sleep.

We have seen already that part of the task of learning to be a parent is finding out when to provide stimulus, and of what kind, and when to withhold stimulus. I watched one very anxious mother with her baby in her arms during and after feeds for a period of twelve hours, and discovered that each time her baby drifted off after a satisfying feed she started to talk to him and twitch the muscles of her shoulders and arms in a quite unconscious attempt to wake him up. She was afraid to let her baby go. When we talked about it I learned that her friend had had a cot death recently and she was anxious lest he should die in his sleep.

There may be less dramatic explanations for some other women behaving in the same way. Another mother with whom I sat for a series of feeds was also in effect saying to her baby 'Look! Here I am! I'm your mother!' and jerking her baby awake. As we talked about it it became clear that she had not yet come to terms with the fact that the baby was outside her, and no longer a part of her in the same intimate way that she was when she was deep inside her body. She felt diminished, nothing, without the baby. Every time people asked about the baby she was reminded that she was a separate entity and felt terribly forlorn. She was only really happy when her baby was breastfeeding.

But even more frequently, mothers prevent their babies from sleeping through muscle tensions and inflection of the voice because they are rushed and anxious to go to a party, finish the housework, write a thesis, paint a picture, cook a meal or do anything rather than sit feeding a baby! Babies pick up such messages with an almost extrasensory perception. The more concerned a mother is to finish the feed and get going, the more likely it is that the baby will not settle down.

It is worth discovering what you do when you are eagerly anticipating some activity which involves the baby being asleep, and finding out how your body reacts. The section on Stanislavski relaxation using 'body memory' and 'emotion memory' in *The Experience of Childbirth*[10] may help you do this. You will find, for example, that there are special patterns of muscle contraction and that your breathing rate is changed. It is important to learn how to relax when feeding the baby, if only to avoid frequent cancellation of social plans!

Many women say that it is exactly the same too when they are planning on making love. The baby senses the excitement and stays awake!

The baby's ability to decode these non-verbal messages which are conveyed unconsciously by the adult body is one explanation for the fact that the 'colicky' baby nearly always has a fussing or crying time in the evening, starting when both parents may want to have some time for themselves.

10. Difficulties

My husband sails for pleasure. I have always been amazed at how sailing, particularly the important going in and out of a crowded port, seems to be a series of crises and yet sailors enjoy it. I sit in the cabin trying to read (or write) a book and hear the continuous thudding of feet overhead, instructions to let this out, coil that, throw out something, bring in this, furl, tighten, mind the –! Parenthood is the same, and especially the going out of port after the birth of a baby, but some mothers and fathers take to it with more relish than others who are unable to face recurrent crises with the same gusto.

Only very rarely does a baby 'make no difference' to a couple's life together, even though this may have been what they determined beforehand. Where both parents are focused on the baby and get pleasure from leading baby-centred lives during the first months, they may not notice how much everything about their existence has changed, and so may underestimate the dramatic change of direction in their lives. Where the mother alone is struggling to maintain a semblance of normality and to continue as before the baby came, but does not have her husband's cooperation, she is fighting a battle which she is bound to lose.

Especially when a couple have put off having a baby until it seemed the 'logical' next step, they may find the shift of focus on to one small human being, and the resulting gulf that separates them from their friends who do not have babies and so cannot understand and make the necessary concessions to their state, intolerable and destructive of the sense of personal worth. This leads to conflict between husband and wife, as each projects on to the other an inner anger at not being able to cope.

Most women face some difficulties when they breastfeed,

especially at first. Even one who thoroughly enjoys feeding her two-month-old baby may have encountered all sorts of challenges when he was still only a few weeks old which at the time made her feel that she was not going to succeed, and that even if she did she was a failure as a mother and had started the baby's life off in such misery that he would be psychologically ruined!

The one thing essential for happy breastfeeding is a large dose of confidence in oneself. This is what the peasant mother has who feeds her babies so easily: complete faith that she is doing the natural and obvious thing in the natural and obvious way. As a result she handles her baby confidently, even if this is quite different from how experts would do it. That apparently simple task is composed of quite complicated sequences. As skill has developed, however, the expertise has become caught up in the flowing movement of the whole activity.

Anybody handling and feeding a baby for the first time tends to make awkward, clumsy movements, because each manipulation has to be worked out and practised before it too becomes part of a rhythmic total activity. This is why it is fatal to be in a position where you feel you have to 'put on a performance' or demonstrate that you possess a skill, and why I believe it is best to get to know your baby, make your own mistakes, and work out your own way of doing things, in private, where just father and mother together can learn how to respond to their baby's needs and how to cope with difficulties.

The flow between mother and baby which is an essential part of spontaneous good mothering is what we are aiming at in 'mothercraft', It is what all advice and help ought to be trying to create. I believe very strongly that any advice, however good it seems, that saps a woman's faith in herself and her ability to mother her baby, and for that matter the father's ability to care for his child, is counterproductive.

But, of course, there *are* skills in breastfeeding, and every difficulty a new mother encounters has probably been met by many mothers before her. Solutions can be suggested, often slightly different ways of handling, or a more sensitive, generous way of responding to the baby rather than trying to obey the instructional manuals to the letter. When skills seem not to work it is often because a mother has been confused by advice coming from many different quarters and has been trying first one thing and then another, without the confidence to try any one approach long enough. The suggestions that I have to make in the following pages are not made as the *only* solution to a common difficulty. Sometimes I have suggested several alternative courses of action. The important thing is that you decide what *you* want to do and having made your choice give it a chance to work.

Here are some of the main difficulties and suggestions as to what to do about them. Some are mainly concerned with the mother, some mainly with the baby, but most concern the interaction between the two of them, even if at first sight they appear to be problems with the breasts or the way the baby sucks or the milk supply. This is because the mother and breastfed baby are in a nursing partnership which is essentially a symbiotic relationship. The baby needs the mother, but the mother whose breasts are full and who longs to give milk also needs the baby. The two are interdependent. When there are difficulties the solutions, more often than not, lie in the interaction between them.

We have seen already, in Chapter 8, that babies have personalities. This is why what works for you may not work for another mother who has a quite different baby. But some of the difficulties encountered are at least in some respects mechanical. These are what we shall be looking at in this chapter.

AFTER-PAINS

As you first breastfeed you may be disconcerted to experience pain in the uterus remarkably like labour contractions. This is because oxytocin is liberated in your blood stream by the baby's sucking, and it makes the uterine muscle contract. When the uterus is approximately the size and shape that it was before the pregnancy this will stop. Suckling often achieves this effect in two or three days.

Treatment

Welcome these contractions, drop your shoulders, and do slow breathing, allowing the abdominal wall to expand on the breath in and then very slowly sink in again on a long breath out. Slow breathing can be done quietly through the nose without worrying anyone who is near by. This is really better than taking painkillers, which, even though present in your milk in small doses, might make the baby less alert just at a time when she is learning important things about the world around her and sending out important messages to you.

ENGORGED BREASTS

When transitional milk begins to come in on the third or fourth day after delivery many women become *engorged*, and the breasts get swollen, hot, lumpy and heavy, with the nipples gradually receding into the breast tissue. Then it is difficult for the baby to get a grip on the nipple with her mouth, even though the milk is there. This problem is very easily dealt with.

If you have been putting the baby to the breast regularly to suck colostrum, it is unlikely that your breasts get time to become severely engorged, unless it has occurred overnight when the baby was given a bottle feed. This is one reason why if the hospital will consent to let the baby come to you whenever she cries, day or night, easy breastfeeding can be more speedily established. It is worth discussing this with the paediatrician. If you have your baby at home the problem does not arise.

But if you do get engorged it is essential to act promptly. This is why you need to know yourself what to do, as it may not be convenient to get someone else to help in the middle of the night. Three days after my twins were born I sat talking to my mother for an hour or so. I was feeling well and very happy. As I got up to go back to my room I realized that I could not lift either arm, because I was so engorged. I went straight to a wash-basin and sponged hot water over both breasts until the milk began to flow. Then I suckled both babies. I breastfed them both without any problems for over ten months.

So if you are engorged draw off a little milk until you are comfortable and the nipples stand out so that your baby can grip them. It is usually simpler to do this if you make the breasts warm first, either by lying with a hot water bottle against them, by sponging them with hot water (not just on top, but the sides and underneath as well) or by having a hot bath or shower. If you choose to have a bath kneel so that your breasts hang in the hot water, and you will soon have a luxurious milk bath! If you choose a shower, stand so that the jet of hot water goes straight on to your breasts. This treatment alone may give you immediate relief and you are then ready to feed the baby. If necessary, wake the baby at this point. You need her as much as she needs you.

Breast massage

If you are still uncomfortable you can massage the breasts. This is best done by the mother herself or by her husband, and should not cause pain. In fact, it should be like a caress, a loving, tender action rather than a detached, impersonal task. It can either be done using two hands and massaging with the thumbs of each, or supporting the breast with one hand and massaging with the other. Here are the two methods.

Single hand massage. Cup one hand under the breast and with the palm of the other do a slow, deep circular massage, using a squeezing movement, above and at either side of the breast, including any swollen glandular tissue in the armpits. Then use the edge of this hand to stroke lightly down towards the nipple and continue this all round the upper curve of the breast. There is no need to touch the nipple.

Massage using two hands. Hold the breast with two hands so that the fingers of each meet underneath the breast and the thumbs touch above the nipple and areola. Allow your breast to drop heavily into the hands so that you get a firm package. Now slowly massage with the thumbs down towards the areola, moving down with a sweeping movement to reach the underlying structures, doing this only as firmly as is comfortable, and coming up lightly again. This presses the milk down into the lactiferous ducts.

In Jamaica peasant women massage their breasts in the days after birth using a comb drawn through a bar of very wet soap. It provides gentle, firm rhythmic massage. I find that this *combing the breasts* works well with English mothers too, and show them how to do this if they are having difficulty getting the baby on to the nipple because the breasts are engorged. It is an unconventional approach, but you may be lucky and get a West Indian midwife who remembers seeing mothers doing this at home.

When you have been massaging the breasts for a few minutes the chances are that drops of milk have appeared at the nipple, and you may even have a fine stream of milk squirting out. But you can now do something more to produce milk in a steady jet. This is *hand expression*. Expression also can be done with one hand or two.

Single hand expression. Support the breast with the hand at the side, thumb half way up, fingers underneath, and sweep the thumb down towards the areola with a gentle movement. Just as the thumb touches the outer circumference of the areola press it in, and squeeze up at the same time with the fingers lying under the breast. It may help to picture 'fifteen to twenty "balloons" full of milk radially around the breast'.[1] Again, do not touch the nipple, or you will shut off the ducts. Milk will stream out. Pick up your baby, make yourself comfortable and put her to the breast.

Expression using both hands. With the hands in the same position as for massaging with both hands, press the thumbs down on the outer edge of the areola so that the nipple stands out more, release them a little, press again, and continue rhythmically in this way. Milk will spurt from the nipple. Avoid squeezing the nipple or it will close the ducts. Now feed your baby.

If you are expressing in order to relieve engorgement, stop as soon as you feel comfortable. The more you stimulate the breasts by expressing milk the more milk you will produce.

Once you are able to get the milk flowing and the nipple erect, wake your baby and feed her.

When you have finished a feed you can use a cold compress against the breasts for comfort; some women find that ice tied in a nappy is soothing, or a soft cushion-type picnic freezing pack kept in the fridge so that it acts as an ice pack. Frozen hard, it will be like a brick; about half frozen is ideal. Massage and heat *before* feeds and ice afterwards is an effective treatment for engorged breasts. Do not do anything that does not increase comfort. Let your feelings guide you. Some people believe heat is the correct treatment, others that ice or cold compresses are the only answer. If you do what relieves pain best in your case, you cannot go wrong.

SECONDARY ENGORGEMENT

When the baby first sleeps through the night you may suddenly discover that you have painfully engorged breasts in the morning, even if you have avoided engorgement before. The same thing can occur if you want to leave the baby for a long period and go out leaving a bottle of expressed breast milk for the feed.

Treatment

Lean over a wash-basin and sponge hot water on the breasts, kneel with the breasts suspended in a hot bath, or sit with a towel under your breasts and hot face flannels on them, and use gentle pressure of both hands to start the milk spurting out. As soon as you can put the baby to the breast, do so. As she feeds, press with the palm of one hand on different areas under the circumference of the breast, especially over any parts which are reddened and tender, where milk has collected.

THE BABY CANNOT GET A GOOD GRIP
ON THE NIPPLE

This may either be because the breast is engorged, or because the nipple is flat or inverted. If the nipple does not stick out sufficiently because the surrounding breast is swollen and full you will need to express some milk before the baby comes to the breast, and may find this easier to do if you rest a hot flannel or nappy on the breast first or squeeze comfortably hot water over it. Massage and expression is described on page 107.

Whereas the usual nipple stands out when it has been stimulated by touch, the inverted nipple retracts. In fact it is more like a dimple than a nipple. A baby can suck on a dimpled nipple and will gradually draw it out, but it is more difficult and you will need to have patience. At first the baby will have to get most of the areola in her mouth as if it were the nipple. Most babies soon get the hang of this provided they are not offered the easy stimulus of a bottle teat. In this case too, it is important to give frequent, fairly short feeds, so that the baby does not tire, nor get so hungry in between feeds that she comes to the breast in an over-excited state.

In between feeds it is a good idea to wear a Woolwich nipple shield or 'shell'. Woolwich shields can be bought at chemists shops. The pressure of the bra on the nipple shield eases the nipple out. Some women find that it helps to wear this from the seventh month of pregnancy. Milk will leak out into the shield and should be thrown away, as the warmth of your body could nourish bacteria. Get ready to feed the baby before you remove the nipple shield as the nipple will continue to hold its shape for a little while and you may be able to slip the baby on the breast while it is still sticking out quite well.

BABIES USED TO BOTTLE FEEDING

Sometimes a baby who has been bottle-fed, especially through a teat with a large hole in it, has learned how to control the flow of milk by pushing her tongue up against the teat. If she does this when put to the breast she will not be able to suck and will become very frustrated, since the sucking action at the breast is different from that from a bottle.

Treatment

You will need great patience. She will probably get very bothered at the breast. Wait until she has her mouth wide open, which is likely to happen soon as she will start to cry, and then slip the nipple firmly in, making sure that it reaches the back of her palate. Cradle her head in the crook of your arm firmly so that she does not pull away from the nipple and start pushing it with her tongue again. Stay calm and the let-down reflex will soon occur; once she finds that milk comes this way she will know how to suckle.

SORE NIPPLES

Sore nipples are probably one of the most common reasons for women deciding to stop breastfeeding, and most nursing mothers experience some soreness in the first weeks.

Redheads and blondes are especially likely to develop soreness but can condition the nipples in advance by making sure that the nipples are handled and used in love play as described on page 44.

Treatment

If you get a sore nipple make sure that you are getting the baby fixed on the breast. The major cause of soreness is not getting enough of the areola as well as the nipple into the baby's mouth, with the result that the baby drags on the nipple stem. The art of fixing is described on page 54.

There is bound to be someone who tells you that you are allowing the baby to suck too much and that that is why you are sore. Limiting sucking, far from preventing nipple soreness, can actually cause it. This is because the baby who is taken off the breast after only two or three minutes may be removed before the let-down reflex has had time to occur, especially if the mother is feeling apprehensive, embarrassed or rushed because she is being watched or she must do it in a certain time. Even when the baby is allowed to suck for four or five minutes the let-down may only then have occurred and she is removed just as she has got going. This is hard on the baby as well as the mother's nipples.

Normally some milk stays in the milk pools between feeds. This is the 'foremilk'. But when a large quantity of milk remains in the ducts and milk pools it causes back-pressure which can block the circulation in the breasts. If this continues for a few days the mother becomes painfully engorged, which makes her even less likely to let down when the baby is put to the breast, and a vicious circle has been created. The more engorged the breast, the more the nipple tends to recede into the surrounding swollen tissues so that the baby cannot get a grip on it and bites on the nipple itself, thus increasing nipple soreness and producing cracks and bleeding. Meanwhile the baby is not being fed, nurses are shaking their heads and the mother is worrying that she will not be able to breastfeed.

To any woman contemplating breastfeeding this must sound horrific. But it need not happen. It is the result of poor management of breastfeeding and is often a direct consequence of bad advice.

Nipple soreness is at its most severe before the let-down reflex has occurred, and then tends to disappear quickly. So it is very important to continue until the reflex occurs *and to go on afterwards*. Once the baby has got into the rhythm of steady sucking you will be able to relax and enjoy the feed even though the first couple of minutes may have been painful. If you are going to put the baby to the breast in the first place it is only fair that you should continue long enough for you both to be able to find the feed a satisfying experience.

As the baby sucks she will draw out and shape the nipple so that it is right for her, and this is particularly important if the mother's nipples were inverted or rather flat beforehand. The nipple, being very pliable, adapts itself beautifully to the baby's mouth and sucking, but this often takes about a week to occur.

As the milk comes in it flows more freely. You will probably find that if you are upset or anxious, and even if you feel that you have to put on a performance for someone who is watching critically, the let-down reflex is delayed. I know someone who could not breastfeed in front of her mother because the let-down was completely inhibited. The baby could get the foremilk that remained in the breast just above the nipple, but after this there was no more, and he began to cry and struggle. But usually as you get to know the baby better and become more familiar with breastfeeding the let-down reflex occurs immediately the baby comes to the breast, and sometimes before.

Human babies seem to be designed like other 'continuous sucking' mammals. This does not mean that they literally suck non-stop, although sometimes it feels like that, but that they enjoy being held close and feeding whenever they seek the nipple. Clock-watching or trying to follow somebody else's instructions does not fit the baby's needs and is also hard on your nipples.

If you discover that your let-down reflex comes slowly, and especially if you find that this upsets the baby, it is a good idea to stimulate the breast *before* the feed. Provided you give enough stimulus to one breast, the other will follow suit. It is worth spending a little time exploring what kind of touch, and even what thoughts, get your breast responsive and the let-down reflex working.

Heat treatment

Heat assists the let-down reflex. It may be enough to sit or lie with a hot water bottle against your breast or to sponge it with hot water.

Breast massage

See page 107. Follow this with *hand expression* (see page 108) until drops of milk appear at the nipple.

Going topless

Sore nipples are best treated by allowing them to dry in the air after feeds — avoiding both the use of soap when washing and also plastic-lined nipple pads which tend to keep the nipples damp — and if possible sunbathing topless. Even if it is cold you may be able to do some of the housework topless. If this cannot be arranged, the heat from an electric light bulb provides comforting warmth, or you can use a sunlamp if you are very careful. Make sure that you are four feet away from it, protect your eyes and start with only thirty seconds exposure.

Avoid wearing nylon or synthetic fabrics next to your breasts if you can. A cotton nursing bra is better than a nylon one, at least until the nipples have healed.

Mini-sauna

La Leche mothers in Denver, Colorado, have devised a mini-Sauna using a table lamp without its shade, and a flexible carboard tube.[2] The tube of cardboard must be large enough to hold your breast and should be about the length of your forearm. (If it is too short you can burn your breast.) Fix it with sticky tape, or even rubber bands will do. At one end of the cardboard cut a hole about 2 × 3 inches so that it can slot over a 75–100 watt electric bulb. Slot the cardboard over the bulb before you switch the lamp on, sit or stand at a height so that the bulb is level with your breast, and then switch the lamp on and put the breast with the sore nipple in at the other end of the tube. The nipple is soothed by the warm, dry air circulating around it. Three minutes is ample time at first, and you can do this as often as you wish. Do not answer the phone without switching the lamp off first, as the cardboard may get too hot and burn. Always switch it off when you have finished the sauna.

Creams

A cream or oil or other treatment to nourish or protect the skin may help. Pure lanolin can be useful. Cetavlex is antiseptic, Massé cream is lanolin-based and Kamillosan contains a sandwich of three kinds of oil with camomile. Rotersept, although it sounds like a lawnmower, is an efficient spray. You may prefer to ask your chemist to make up a mixture of almond oil 27·5, arachis oil 27·5 and hamamelis water 27·5, or to get calendula cream from a homoeopathic chemist. You may be allergic to any of these, and should do a patch test on your inside elbow to see if it causes any reddening first of all. Apply the cream or oil *around* the nipple, not over the tip where the openings to the milk ducts could be partially blocked with heavy applications of ointment.

Other things you can do

Give the baby the nipple which is less sore first. As she sucks milk will probably start to spurt out of the sore nipple, so relieving the tension. She will also be less urgently hungry when she gets to the second breast and so will not grip so tightly. The chances are, too, that you will be less tense by the time she is feeding well and this makes any discomfort much easier to bear.

A hungry baby, especially one who has been kept crying while waiting for a feed, feeds as if she is attacking the nipple. It helps to feed more often, before her hunger is acute. If your baby sucks very strenuously and tends to get cross and fight the breast because the let-down does not come quickly enough lift her before she is fully awake whenever possible. That way, the feed starts as a pleasant surprise for her instead of being something she is actively seeking and seeming desperate about. You are more likely to be relaxed and as your baby wakes and sucks the let-down will occur.

When taking the baby off the breast always break the suction by depressing and so dimpling the breast margin or slipping a finger in her mouth and between the gums. *Never* just pull!

Nipple shields

If you have a sore nipple, healing is taking place slowly, and you flinch as you put the baby to the breast you may like the idea of a nipple shield. These work well for some people, not at all for others. When there is a crack in the nipple at the point where it joins the areola, a nipple shield sometimes presses on just that area and causes more pain.

The best nipple shields are very soft and flexible. The Natural Nursing Shield is made of red rubber and looks like a Mexican hat. It has a small teat (the crown of the hat) through which the baby obtains the milk. It is obtainable through John Bell and Croydon and from The National Childbirth Trust, 9 Queensborough Terrace, London, W2. Soak it in Milton solution after a feed and then let it dry in the air.

As soon as you feel you can try the baby on the breast again without using the shield, do so, as the immediate contact between the baby's mouth and your skin will further stimulate the milk supply.

Tea-strainer protectors

Buy small plastic strainers, cut off the handles and insert over the nipples under the bra.[3] This allows air to circulate round the nipples while you are dressed. (Not recommended for party wear!)

Your doctor

Many doctors suggest that mothers put the baby on the bottle if they develop sore nipples. It is as well to be prepared for this unless you know in advance that he or she is experienced in giving support to breastfeeding mothers. The doctor may believe that you are in effect asking permission to stop breastfeeding, and this is certainly the reason why some women seek advice. So it helps to know in your own mind what you really want first of all and, if you intend to continue breastfeeding, to make this clear.

A mother told a group of nursing students, 'Try to imagine

how a young bride would feel if her doctor told her to forget about trying to achieve a satisfying sexual relationship with her husband, because it doesn't really matter' . . .⁴

A RED PATCH ON THE BREAST, POSSIBLE SLIGHTLY RAISED TEMPERATURE

This is a blocked milk duct, and is almost invariably a result of stasis. It tends to occur when the breast has been insufficiently emptied, clothes are constricting and arm movements restricted, and, as we have already seen when talking about the baby, when a small segment of the breast is revealed at which the baby can feed, while the rest of the breast remains tucked away with clothing and your arms pressing on it. If there is also a crack in the nipple which has allowed infection to enter it can be the forerunner of mastitis, so prompt treatment is necessary.

Treatment

Friends may say 'take it easy', not realizing that it is taking it easy which is most likely to lead to stasis. The worst thing you can do is to stop putting the baby to that breast and lie in bed or sit in front of the TV set.

Constriction may also result from too tight a bra, especially if the cup is too small. It is important to see that a bra does not compress the breasts when they are at their fullest just before a feed.

My own observation is that the red patch often develops in the outer lower quadrant of one breast, at the point which is gripped by one's arms when lying in bed or sitting around. Continued feeding whenever the baby wants to suckle from that side and some exercise can help considerably. This should involve energetic arm movements: polishing or scrubbing a floor on all fours, washing and wringing out nappies by hand and squeezing every last drop of water out of them, a fast game of tennis, badminton or squash, swimming or even (if you are in the right place for it) skiing. This may sound harsh treatment for a woman who is already rather feverish and in some pain, but activity will help to relieve the milk blockage, and the mother may notice that milk starts to flow from the affected breast.

Women in peasant communities do not seem to be troubled by this kind of thing and one reason may be because they continue with their work in the house, without modern equipment, sweeping floors, scouring pots, rubbing the linen on stones down by the stream, and may also labour in field or garden. We tend to ignore the value of physical activity of this kind and think of breastfeeding as something special that a woman does which requires a protected environment. But the very measures introduced to try and make breastfeeding easier may actually make it more difficult for her because they result in immobilization and thus produce stasis.

A SHINY, HOT RED PATCH ON THE BREAST AND A RAISED TEMPERATURE OF 104° OR MORE — MASTITIS

An inflamed area on the breast and a raised temperature suggests that you have sporadic mastitis. When this occurs it does so between two and six weeks after the birth and develops in the inter-lobar tissues. *It is not a breast abscess.* Mastitis is much more common than an abscess and a good deal milder, but nevertheless can be extremely uncomfortable. The red patch is extremely tender and you feel as if you were going down with flu. It may follow from untreated blocked ducts, and the bug concerned is usually *Staphylococcus aureus* which does not cause any illness in the baby. In fact, it may have been picked up from the baby's oral cavity and nose in the first place. It is unlikely to lead to an abscess *if you continue to breastfeed.*

Treatment

The most important aspect of treatment is to keep the milk flowing at frequent intervals, with regular nursing (every two to three hours if the baby is happy with this), and hot face flannels or nappies wrung out in hot water and applied over the sore area. This ensures the reduction of congestion in the affected breast. You are much more likely to develop an abscess if you stop using the breast.

Mastitis is speedily treated with penicillin or other antibiotics. You can continue feeding whilst on antibiotics, though the baby's motions may be loose. The infection is usually cleared up in a couple of days.

However, broad-spectrum antibiotics in particular have what Waltar Whittlestone calls 'a devastating effect' on the bacterial flora of the baby's gut, since they kill lactic-acid-producing organisms which protect against infection.[5] An alternative method of treatment is based on that sometimes used with cows, who also get mastitis.

A treatment which has been demonstrated in cattle to be just as effective as antibiotics involves the use of a high dose of oxytocin followed by massage and complete milking out. Translated to the human scene, this would involve the use of oxytocin nasal spray [you will have to ask your doctor to prescribe this] the suckling of the healthy gland and the complete milking out with a suitable breast pump of the infected one. This process sweeps the infecting organisms from the secretory tissue and enables the natural protective mechanism to finally gain the upper hand.[6]

This treatment may need to be repeated every three or four hours until the temperature is normal and the redness disappears. It can also be tried without the use of oxytocin.

In one study acute sporadic mastitis was diagnosed in sixty-one of 2,534 nursing mothers. The most usual time for this condition to develop was five or six weeks after delivery. Four women suffered from it more than once.[7] Three of these women, all of whom had decided to stop breastfeeding, developed breast abscesses. Doctors often advise mothers to stop breastfeeding if they get mastitis, without realizing that it is likely to encourage abscess formation and without understanding the emotional effect of sudden weaning on mother and child.

EPIDEMIC MASTITIS

This is a hospital disease which can occur in those hospitals where babies are kept in nurseries. The baby brings the organisms from the nursery in its nose.

The staphylococci responsible may be resistant to penicillin. The treatment is as for sporadic mastitis, except that hospital staff will take a culture of your milk and may want you to discontinue breastfeeding from that side until the bacteria count is within safe limits. It is important to keep the breast as empty as possible by regular pumping with an electric breast pump.

There is a strong case for asking if the baby can remain with you instead of going back to the nursery, and to request a private room if one is available, where you can both be together. Failing this, home is better than hospital. You will need someone to look after you as you should stay in bed, and the community midwife will call at least once a day to help. The hospital may let you have an electric pump to take home with you. If not, you can hire one through the National Childbirth Trust, 9 Queensborough Terrace, London, W2.

INADEQUATE MILK SUPPLY

By far the most common reason for not having enough milk is that the breast is insufficiently stimulated to produce more milk. Milk is made on a demand and supply system, and unless there is frequent stimulus the supply tails off. Anxiety can inhibit the let-down reflex so that although milk is there you cannot release it. Perhaps this is why mothers are so often told that they need more rest when they are not producing enough milk. But if you are lying in bed worrying about not having sufficient milk or about a toddler who is being cared for by someone else, you are still unlikely to make more milk. I believe that physical rest alone is not helpful and that the reasons for emotional turmoil need to be understood. Sometimes chemical toxicants are reducing the milk supply, as you can see in Chapter 13. The most common

pharmacological cause for a reduced milk supply is the contraceptive pill.

Treatment

It is extremely tiring for both mother and baby to have very
lengthy feeds in a desperate attempt to make more milk.
It is much better to have frequent feeds and to keep these as
short as the baby wants them. The number or frequency of
feeds that any other woman's baby has is irrelevant to your
own baby's needs. Sometimes the baby wants to stay at the
breast and likes to suckle intermittently, but is not really
feeding. Comfort sucking of this kind is an important aspect
of breastfeeding but should not be confused with feeding.
Feeding is distinctive because there is a definite pattern of
suck-swallow or if the milk is coming less fast suck-suck-
swallow. It is sometimes helpful to have someone experienced
watch you and the baby to help you see the difference between these activities.

You can usually rely on the baby to regulate the frequency
and timing of feeds. You do not need a clock. Simply feed her
when she asks and stay close enough to her between feeds so
that you are immediately aware when she is stirring and
might be ready for another feed. Then take the opportunity of
offering another feed *even though she is not crying*. A baby
who is allowed to scream before being offered food may be
too tired then to take a full feed.

Night feeding is also important to build up a good milk
supply. Do not allow yourself to be influenced by any mother
boasting about her baby sleeping through the night. Your
breasts need the stimulus if you are to increase the supply.

Anxiety or depression is something which ought to be
discussed between husband and wife together or with someone else you find it easy to talk with. Often there are changes
in the environment that can be made which offer at least a
partial solution. Sometimes it is important for the man to
protect her from people with whom she has an emotionally
fraught relationship, and this may be her own or his mother

or a sister who is going through emotional problems of her
own and has become dependant. If you are bothered by constant visitors or advisors it may be a good idea to put a notice
on the front door for part of the day which states categoric-
ally 'Mother resting'. The father may be able to reorganize
his time so that he takes more responsibility for a toddler or
for dealing with some household tasks on which the mother
cannot concentrate at this stage.

The relaxation learned in pregnancy to prepare for labour
is also very important when breastfeeding. Re-read the
chapter 'Learning Harmony in Labour: Relaxation' in *The
Experience of Childbirth*, and notice particularly tensions in
the shoulders and the back of your neck. Breathe out and
relax! Let the milk flow!

If the pill might be the cause of the trouble discuss what
other contraceptives to use.

There is more about the milk supply, and its relation to the
kind of baby you have, in Chapter 8, and if you are fast
approaching crisis point look up Chapter 11. 'Crisis', and
follow my *twenty-four-hour peak production plan*.

THE BABY HAS NOT GAINED ENOUGH WEIGHT

Breastfed babies do not usually gain weight so rapidly as
bottle-fed babies and norms based on bottle feeding are not
valid. (The baby who was low weight at birth, however, often
gains weight more quickly than the bottle-fed one.)[8] The
breastfed baby regulates both the quantity and the quality of
milk, as we saw in Chapter 2. If your baby is not gaining
weight be sure to have a flexible routine and let her set the
pace for feeding. This may mean putting her to the breast as
many as ten times in the twenty-four hours, especially in the
first ten days of life. If a breastfed baby is fed whenever she
indicates that she wants to suckle it is very unlikely that she
is being underfed.

*The mother whose baby is on a self-regulating scheme of
feeding and who notices that he produces six to eight wet
nappies in every twenty-four hours can forget all about
weighing her child.* General muscle tone, alertness, bright

eyes and vitality are more important than weekly weight gains.

MILK COMING TOO FAST

A baby who is otherwise healthy, but whose stools are green and semi-liquid but are still sweet-smelling, and who is choking during feeds and may be bringing back some milk during and at the end of a feed, is unable to cope with such a fast flow of milk. This happened to one of my twins when I suckled both babies at the same time. The jet of milk could be heard going straight down into her and she had to keep on drawing back to have time to swallow. I found it was better to feed each baby separately so that we could take the feed more slowly.

Treatment

Express a little milk first. If you have a great quantity of milk simple pressure with hands over and under the breast will produce a steady stream. Put the baby to the breast only when this has slowed down a little. Hold the breast with your hand so that pressure is applied just above and below the areola and this will reduce the rate of flow as the baby suckles. Be calm, unhurried and relaxed yourself and talk soothingly to the baby who may be gulping because of a stressful atmosphere. See if it helps to seek privacy and a quiet room for feeding this baby.

THE DIABETIC MOTHER

A diabetic mother can breastfeed. Lactation may in fact reduce her need for insulin. It is important for her to keep in touch with her diabetologist after delivery, whether or not she breastfeeds. In one study of seventeen insulin-dependant diabetic mothers six had an average decrease of insulin dosage of 33 per cent, seven a decrease of 13 per cent and only four needed to have slightly more insulin while they breastfed, which related directly to the increased need for calories.[10] So although you need extra calories to supply milk for your baby you may actually find that the amount of insulin you need falls after delivery. It is unwise to try to lose weight rapidly, and if you want to slim keep in close touch with your doctor about this.

Since you may have been separated from your baby while it was cared for initially in the special care baby unit it is especially important for you to feel that you can breastfeed and have a good start with the feeding relationship.

At the present state of knowledge there is no indication that the milk of the diabetic mother is not perfectly all right for her baby. Levels of insulin in her blood are not very different from those that will be in her blood if she is not diabetic and is producing her own insulin.

Metabolic and hormonal changes after the birth entail an adjustment of insulin, whether or not she is breastfeeding. If she is breastfeeding she needs to increase her calories, since lactation requires several hundred extra calories a day.[11] She should watch her health carefully and if there is no ketonuria or other signs that her diabetes is getting out of hand, and little glycosuria, she can safely breastfeed, but there is usually a time of trial and error to start with when she will need to find out her personal requirements for insulin and calories, and her doctor will help her sort this out.

If she becomes hypoglycaemic she will have bad headaches, shivering, sweating, trembling and palpitations, and all of this will tend to make her anxious and less likely to be able to breastfeed happily. So it is very important that she lives sensibly and cares for her health for the sake of her baby and that her blood and urine glucose levels are tested regularly. If any symptoms of hypoglycaemia occur, make an appointment with the doctor, and meanwhile try reducing the insulin doseage.

Should ketosis develop, which usually occurs after a prolonged period of hypoglycaemia when warning symptoms have been ignored or inadequately treated, she needs an increased insulin dosage, more carbohydrate in her diet and plenty of fluids. Again, make an appointment with the doctor.

The mother's emotional state is also important in the control of diabetes.[12] Anxiety can affect glucose levels and she will do best in a peaceful environment in which she can relate to her baby in her own way and have the satisfaction of feeling that she is giving her baby the best possible food.

11. Crisis

Some of the crises confronted with a new baby can be shattering. It is not just a matter of not being able to breastfeed and having to change to the bottle; sometimes it can feel like an assault on the integrity of the mother's whole personality.

Just one letter of the many hundreds I have had from women seeking help may give an idea of the depths of misery which can be experienced (I have altered it slightly so that the writer cannot be identified):

Please help me. I'm desperate. My new baby started to cry an awful lot when she was five days old and because I was worried that she wasn't getting enough breast milk I gave her a couple of ounces of SMA. Since then she has been getting a small complementary bottle after each feed, so that now she is nearly four weeks old she gets a total of 10 oz. SMA a day. I tried testweighing her after each breastfeed and at no time was I producing more than 60g. (2 oz.).

I am in a highly depressed state. At the end of this week she had only gained 2 oz. which wasn't enough so I have been giving her more bottles. I feel so upset and indecisive. I very much want to be able to feed her completely myself. Somehow my value as a woman seems to depend on it. I felt such a failure with my older child. The hospital where she was born decided that my nipples were too flat so they bottle fed her.

I vaccilate between feeling that breastfeeding my baby is of such great value I ought to try to screw myself up to persisting without the bottles and alternately labelling myself as self-ish for wanting to do it so that I will feel adequate.

Please, oh please, what should I do? I should rewrite this letter, it seems too confusing but I don't think in my present mental state that I could do any better at a second attempt.

One of the first crises may occur when mother and baby are still in hospital and the parents discover that their baby is in special care and being fed in the nursery before the mother's own milk has come in.

LOW BLOOD SUGAR IN THE
LOW-BIRTH-WEIGHT BABY[1]

Some years ago it used to be the practice to leave very small and premature babies without food in the first days after birth because doctors were worried about them vomiting and then inhaling milk into their lungs, and thus choking. As a result some babies lost far too much weight after birth and their blood sugar fell too low. The baby with low blood sugar may sleep peacefully, although symptoms of hypoglycaemia – including jerking and irritability, episodes when the baby turns blue or stops breathing for a few seconds, or convulsions – may occur. Studies have shown that marked hypoglycaemia results in reduced brain development. Paediatricians watch for hypoglycaemia if a baby is of low birth weight, and it is one common reason for hospitals giving babies additional artificial feeds.

The period when this is most likely to occur is on the second and third days of life. So paediatricians may want to give the dysmature baby – a baby who was 'small for dates' and who seems to have suffered from some placental failure to give good nutrition at the end of pregnancy – prophylactic milk feeds before the breast milk comes in and, if the baby has obvious symptoms of hypoglycaemia, additional glucose or fructose straight into the blood stream.

At birth a baby has a level of blood sugar a little below that of the mother's. It then falls in the first twenty-four hours, to rise again to a normal level somewhat lower than that of an adult. The baby who was well nourished in the uterus can cope with this because there are adequate glycogen stores in the liver. The one who was undernourished in the uterus, perhaps because of maternal toxaemia and an underfunctioning placenta, cannot tolerate this drop in blood sugar.

This is very alarming for a mother who wants to give her baby the best start in life and who is longing to breastfeed. But the period during which the low-weight or premature baby is at risk lasts only about twenty-four to thirty-six hours, and the mother who is keen that her baby should only have breast milk can ask that she should be given expressed breast milk from the hospital milk bank. It is often possible to arrange for another breastfeeding mother who has plenty of milk to provide enough for the new baby. The Breastfeeding Promotion Group of the National Childbirth Trust is used to moving quickly to make such arrangements. Ring 01–229 9319 or 9310, the local branch or any antenatal teacher of the National Childbirth Trust.

If only glucose water, not extra milk, is considered necessary for the low-birth-weight baby, this can be given in a spoon, or even a medicine dropper, so that she does not get accustomed to the easy sucking from a bottle, and associates the satisfaction of sucking with the mother's breast only. One difficulty with bottle teats is that they provide a 'super stimulus' to which the baby may respond in place of the mother's nipple. Giving any additional feeds by spoon avoids this problem, and because it takes time means that complements are not given thoughtlessly, 'just in case'.

It is important to stimulate your own milk supply if the baby is in the special care baby unit and especially if she is not sucking strongly, perhaps because she is being adequately fed by bottle or by a tube passed right down into the stomach which saves her the trouble of sucking at all. This is usually easily done with an electric breast pump such as the Egnell pump. Most hospitals have at least one pump, but if your hospital does not have one you can hire one from the NCT. Details of hand-operated pumps which are small and simple to use, and which can be taken wherever you go, are on page 227.

The risk of hypoglycaemia is not an excuse for giving artificial feeds to all newborn babies or for stuffing them full of glucose water. When I looked at what was happening in British maternity hospitals today[2] I discovered that in some units mothers were being told that their babies must have glucose whatever their birth weight and many, quite rightly, objected to this practice. If your baby is considered to need additional feeds and sugar it is reasonable to expect that this should be fully explained to you by the paediatrician, and a good idea to ask to talk to him or her about it. If you know already that you have an 'at risk' baby you will be in a better position to understand why this is being done; if your baby is clearly not 'at risk' you can ask that this should not be done, and if it is hospital policy to give all babies glucose you may choose to discharge yourself and the baby. Community midwives are usually very supportive of the breastfeeding mother and will not suggest that you give your baby anything other than breast milk unless she is not thriving. Most babies do not need anything except their mother's milk.

THE CRISIS OF GOING HOME FROM HOSPITAL

The first crisis which the parents have to handle more or less on their own comes when mother and baby return from hospital. This often coincides with the time, between four and eight days after birth, when the baby needs more milk than before and wakes frequently for feeds. Going home is almost always a crisis for the new mother. It involves a transition from an institutional environment to one where the parents themselves must accept full responsibility for the baby. It also involves a new self-awareness as one gets back into a familiar environment for the first time as a different person, a mother.

Going home coincides with a *peak demand* for feeding on the part of the baby, since days four and five are those in which the baby has used up its initial supplies of fat. The result is often that the baby becomes restless and cries far more than in hospital and that the mother may feel that she has less milk than she had while she was in hospital. It is therefore wise to anticipate that the baby may need more concentrated care and more frequent feeds for twenty-four hours after the return home, and to make provision for it. Some babies are almost continuous feeders at this stage. Others will go for two or three hours between feeds. Some wake several times in the night. Others provide their parents with very welcome sleep by waking only once in the night. The parents cannot dictate the rhythm. All they can do is to adapt to their baby's needs.

Unfortunately this is also often the time when visitors call, and it can be difficult to fit in social contacts with caring for the baby. But the baby must come first. It is also often the time when a woman arranges for her mother or parents-in-law to come to stay, the worst possible time to plan for this. Ideally the first few days after coming out of hospital should be devoted to the creation of the new family, and mother, father and baby should be close together, getting to know each other — best of all, in the same bed.

A 'BABYMOON'

A babymoon is a holiday spent by the new parents with their baby which takes place for the most part in the bedroom. They get in food and drink in advance and make forays to the kitchen, but spend most of the time in bed with their baby. They do not receive visitors, and make it known beforehand that they will be otherwise occupied. They might even put up a notice on the door 'Parents resting'. The only other person who is allowed in is the midwife who pays her daily visit and, if they are fortunate, a cleaning lady or a friend or relative willing to take on this role who washes the dishes and the nappies, but keeps out of their way. Couples in our society need babymoons even more, perhaps, than they need honeymoons. They need a space in their lives when they come to terms with the momentous event which has occurred and can begin to understand their baby's signals. Since the man will have to take time off work the babymoon may only last a few days, but even if it is that brief it can be an important contribution to the psychological well-being of the new family.

In planning ahead for the birth it is a good idea to plan for the babymoon too, and to see that there is food in the store cupboard and perhaps a bottle of wine or two, some luxury items which might normally be considered too expensive, and some candles for creating the right atmosphere. Birth is a celebration!

THE SIX-WEEK CRISIS

The second normal crisis occurs when the baby is five or six weeks old. At about this time most babies have an appetite spurt and need more milk. The only way the milk can be stimulated is by feeding more frequently. Yet the parents are usually hoping that things have 'settled down' by then and are trying to establish rhythms which are compatible with a life-style which is not entirely baby-centred. They want to see something of their friends, to get out a bit together, and also realize that the new grandmothers are wanting to see more of the baby. So the baby's demands often come at a socially inopportune time.

The mother notices that the baby does not settle well after feeds, wakes crying again after dozing for half an hour or so and chews her fist in between suckling times. She is afraid that she is losing her milk. Many women give up breastfeeding at about this time because they discover that their breasts are not as full and firm as they were in the earlier weeks of breastfeeding and believe that they have no milk. But the engorgement of the first postpartum weeks is a sign that the milk-giving breasts are getting into working order, and is not a necessary concomitant of adequate lactation. As the breasts adjust to feeding they get softer and smaller again, though they vary at different times of the day, and a lactating woman usually wakes in the morning with swelling breasts. Her milk is there, however, and is replenished, provided the baby suckles, throughout the twenty-four hours, not just in the early morning.

The more often the baby suckles, the more milk will be produced. Frequency of feeds is more important than long suckling. The baby gets most of the milk in the first few minutes at the breast anyway.

It is often at this crisis that the mother is recommended to give an occasional bottle. The problem here is that if the baby is given other food suckling at the breast is bound to be reduced and milk production, instead of being increased, will begin to fall off.

Instead the mother might consider my twenty-four-hour peak production plan.

THE TWENTY-FOUR-HOUR PEAK PRODUCTION PLAN

If a mother is able to devote herself almost entirely to her baby's needs and respond to each and every signal from the baby that she wants to suckle, there will be a rapid and marked increase in the production of breast milk. Sometimes it does not even take this long. But it is sensible to plan for a twenty-four-hour period set aside for this purpose.

This means that the couple should discuss together arrangements and the husband may need to protect his wife from other commitments and from unwanted visitors at this time. It is sometimes difficult to arrange when there are other children; extra help in the house may be required, or someone who will take a toddler out to the park. The husband is often the best person to take over responsibility for older children, and this may be easier to arrange at the week-end.

The mother and baby need a *sanctuary* in order to cope with this crisis. The best one is usually the mother's own bed. The husband can see to it that such a sanctuary is provided and that it is a protected environment for the nursing couple.

The baby will probably need feeding every two or three hours, and the stimulus provided by suckling as frequently as this is enough to get the milk flowing freely. If the baby is drowsy and does not wake after three hours she can be gently roused. Even if she does not wake completely at that point she will probably suckle a little and give the breasts further stimulus.

During this time it is important to have enough fluids. If you have become tense about feeding, wine or beer may help you relax, as well as providing fluid. You will probably feel thirsty when putting the baby to the breast, so have a jug of water or juice on the bedside table. You may also appreciate frequent pots of tea and milk drinks. There is no advantage in drinking to excess. Research shows that mothers who drink large amounts of fluid because they feel they *ought* to, produce less milk than those who drink just as much as they want. But the breastfeeding mother is naturally thirsty. Let your thirst guide you.

When mothers ring me to say that they have been advised to put the baby on the bottle because they do not have enough milk I usually suggest that we try my twenty-four-hour approach first if they can spare the time and would like to. Sometimes the mother has become so anxious that it seems better to ask her if she would prefer to do this at my home. What is happening then is that another woman, one with experience, acts to contain the situation and provide the sanctuary.

At this crisis point there is a role for a person who is able to mother the mother. Some writers believe that all new mothers need mothering. Dana Raphael,[3] writing of the 'doula' in societies where a female member of the extended family or another woman in the community moves in to give support to the lactating woman after delivery, asserts that breastfeeding women in our own society too need to be pampered and cared for by someone acting in the role of a mother to the new mother. I believe that many new mothers resent mothering and want to strike out on their own and do things *their* way. They welcome the support of other mothers with whom they can share experiences and enjoy being in a network of women in the role of sisters. But they do not appreciate anybody who mothers them. Once a crisis is reached, however, such as the one at six weeks, a proportion of them need a different kind of emotional support, and for a limited time mothering the mother is an appropriate kind of help. Even so, this must be done unobtrusively, and the other women must support the new mother in establishing her independence and in growing away from the need for help of this kind. This means that anyone who offers support must be free of any need for others to be emotionally dependent on her; her capacity to mother must come out of her own full-ness of living.

The person who helps should also be able to give them-selves without placing on the mother a burden of gratitude or of responsibility to succeed at all costs. There is a tempta-tion in any counselling to give so much that the client experiences guilt if she cannot live up to one's expectations and is then resentful of the amount of one's gift. The breast-feeding counsellor may also exhaust her own inner resources if she pours all her energy into each helping task. Anna Freud has said that it is important 'not to *lose* oneself, but to *lend* something of oneself'.⁴ If the helping person is able to do that she is then enriched every time the one who is helped becomes strong enough not to need her any more.

A CRACKED NIPPLE

Any of the difficulties described in Chapter 10 may amount to a crisis. A sore nipple may, for example, develop a crack in it after five to eight days of feeding, and this is acutely painful. As the baby first fixes on the breast there is a sharp, shooting pain which makes you wince. It can be alarming to see milk emerging streaked with blood and if you did not realize that this is what happens when a nipple is cracked you might think that something more drastic had occurred in the depths of the breast.

The treatment for this is exactly the same as for sore nipples, but if this is not sufficiently effective to clear it up you may prefer to take the baby off that side for twenty-four to thirty-six hours and continue feeding during that time from one breast only. There will be quite enough for the baby if you feed on demand. But do not leave the breast with the cracked nipple to become engorged. Express the milk, either by hand or with a pump. You can give the baby this milk in a teaspoon. Use a large towelling nappy as much of it will not go inside her mouth. It is easiest for her to taste and swallow it if you insert the spoon just inside the corner of her mouth. Any drops of blood in the milk will not hurt her. (Masai warriors drink the blood of their cows to give them extra strength!)

BREAST ABSCESS

This is an acute infection in the milk ducts leading to a pus-filled lump which, if it cannot be cleared up with antibiotics, has to be surgically drained. It is likely to occur in women who have stopped breastfeeding because they have developed mastitis (see page 110).

Surprisingly, it is possible for a woman to continue breast-feeding with an abscess if she wants to, even if she needs an operation. There is no evidence that the baby suffers any harm from it. Immunological substances in the milk probably protect the baby from the staphyloccoci causing the abscess. But even if you do not want to do this, you can continue feeding the baby from the other side and pump the milk from the affected breast and throw it away until the infection has cleared up, when you can go back to feeding from that side too.

NO MILK!

It is very rare indeed for a woman to produce no milk at all. I used to believe that it could not happen until I met a mother whose baby was about six weeks old and who longed to breastfeed, but who had got off to a bad start in a hospital where she became anxious about a milk supply that was obviously coming in very slowly, and was weeping over her baby at every feed. She was advised to put the baby on the bottle and the drops of milk she had been able to produce at the nipple disappeared completely, and frequent suckling in a relaxed atmosphere failed to initiate re-lactation.

It is usually not difficult to re-lactate at any time during the baby's first three months of life, and this is often done by mothers in Africa who have to leave their babies for treatment in hospital for a period of weeks. The baby should be put to the breast as frequently as possible and topped up with formula until the time comes, sometimes after only three or four days, when each suckling is clearly producing enough milk to keep the baby satisfied until she is picked up again when she stirs. Suckling about every two hours during the day (and less often at night) may be necessary for two or three weeks.

A woman who fears that she has no milk should follow the suggestions on page 132 in the twenty-four-hour peak pro-duction plan. She will usually be pleasantly surprised.

Inability to lactate does not mean that the baby cannot be fed at the breast. The Lact-aid Nursing Supplementer provides the baby with formula or human milk from a donor which is sucked through a fine tube placed beside the mother's nipple so that the baby needs to suckle at the breast in order to obtain the milk. This usually leads to lactation because the stimulus to the breast, combined with the woman's knowledge that her baby is being nourished, results in milk production and let-down.[5] The woman whom I have already mentioned who did not lactate decided that this was the next best thing to true breastfeeding, and succeeded in suckling her baby for the first year of life.

The apparatus is lightweight so is worth getting from the USA if you cannot get it immediately from La Leche in the UK. The kit includes an instruction book by Jimmie Lynne Avery, who breastfed two adopted babies in this way, a roll of 100 bags of 4 oz. capacity, a funnel, and rather fiddly tabs for attaching to the bra. An optional extra is a neck cord intended to be worn at night or at other times when the mother is wearing no bra, but this is usually easier to use all be ordered to come by airmail.

THE MOTHER BECOMES ILL

If the mother runs a fever the milk supply may be diminished, but plenty of fluids and frequent suckling will help her and her baby through this crisis. Sometimes she desperately needs a night's sleep, for either physical or emotional reasons. She should express her breast milk either by hand if she is skilled at this, or with a breast pump, the bung and breast cup of which have been sterilized in Milton solution, into a plastic container which has been Milton sterilized, heat dried in a dishwasher, or rinsed in boiling water. It can be safely stored in the fridge for twenty-four hours if necessary. A small hand pump is extremely useful in such situations and there are some excellent ones on the American market. Sears Roebuck make one which works by pressing a rubber balloon in a rhythm which imitates the baby's sucking action, the milk being collected in a feeding bottle with a wide top. In the UK the Egnell and Kaneson pumps are obtainable through the NCT.[6]

In an emergency you can use a large fruit-juice jar (which has a mouth wide enough to contain the nipple and areola) to construct a home-made pump.[7] Glass kitchen containers for herbs, rice, etc. may also be the right size, but check first that they will take boiling water. Breastfeeding mothers in Denver, Colorado, discovered this method. Wash and rinse the jar carefully. Put on oven gloves and fill the jar with water which has boiled and allowed to cool for a minute. Put the kettle on again as you will need more boiling water for pumping the second breast. Pour the hot water out of the jar and wipe its mouth round with a face flannel wrung out in cold water to speed the cooling of the top while the lower part stays hot. Take off the oven gloves. When the mouth of the jar feels comfortably hot to your inside wrist, wet your breast with warm water and leaning over the jar let the nipple and areola fall into the mouth of the jar so that there is an airtight seal. Use the damp, cool face flannel to wipe round the base of the jar. As the hot air cools slowly it contracts and produces a gentle, stimulating vacuum suction. Avoid wrapping the jar completely in a cold cloth or the cooling will take place too quickly and create uncomfortable suction. Gently press over the fifteen to twenty milk-filled 'balloons' radially around the breast and milk will stream out. Whenever you want to stop, put a finger between the breast and the mouth of the jar to break the suction. Repeat the process for the other breast.

If a mother has to go into hospital her breastfed baby should go with her, and the pair should have a private room or amenity bed. It is outrageous that any hospital should separate a mother and baby because the mother needs treatment which can be given only in hospital. A woman who is feeling weak or drowsy can breastfeed perfectly well if her husband or someone else holds the baby at her breast. But if she is coming round from an anaesthetic she should not breastfeed until the anaesthesia is out of her blood stream and she is feeling reasonably alert. If there is time to plan ahead breast milk can be expressed in advance and stored in the fridge or frozen for later use. If not, a donor mother may be able to provide breast milk over a short period. Contact the National Childbirth Trust. Or the baby can be given a bottle of formula for one feed. Following this, the mother's breasts will probably fill up with milk and become uncomfortable even though she is ill or recovering from an operation, and she needs her baby as much as the baby needs her. Drugs can usually be selected which do not contaminate breast milk, or do so to a minimal degree. There is information about this in Chapter 13.

EMERGENCY ACTION WHEN A FEED OR FEEDS MUST BE MISSED

If for social reasons, or in a family crisis, a woman has to be away from her baby during a time when she may need to suckle, a breast pump can be used to collect milk sufficient to cover this period, or a bottle or two of formula can be given. If you have a freezer there is an advantage in storing some frozen expressed breast milk in case an emergency of this kind may crop up. For the same reason it is useful for a baby to get accustomed to the occasional use of a bottle for a feed so that whatever happens the mother need not worry that her baby might not be fed. There is no reason why this should contain artificial milk and there are strong reasons for giving only breast milk if possible. Offering a bottle once every week or ten days keeps the baby accustomed to the idea that milk can come in this way too. But *it often does not work if the mother gives the bottle*, since the baby associates her with breastfeeding. So the father or a friend should take over for this feed.

The mother may find herself becoming engorged if she does not express some milk regularly at the times when the baby was likely to be fed. If she must be away from her baby for more than twenty-four hours and wants to keep up her milk supply she needs to find a quiet place where she can express milk equivalent in amount to that which the baby was taking, and can usually do this more efficiently using a breast pump than by hand expression.

Some writers and breastfeeding counsellors suggest that it

is useful to be able to express milk so that feeds can be missed for the mother to get out of the home and away from her baby to fulfil social engagements. Each woman must decide for herself how important this is for her, and only she knows. But it is usually possible to carry on an active social life and take the baby as well. I feel strongly that if it is not, we should change society, rather than break up the partnership between the nursing mother and her baby for trivial reasons.

It is a different matter if the mother is working outside the home and cannot take her baby with her. Here again, we should be working to change society so that the needs of mothers and babies are catered for. But in the meantime it may be necessary to evolve techniques of organization so that breastfeeding takes place during the time one is with the baby and bottles of expressed breast milk or formula are given at other times. This is possible if the mother is prepared to use the night for feeding. On the other hand, if she is at full stretch in her work she may find this too tiring.

THE BABY GETS ILL

Completely breastfed babies are far less likely to get ill than artificially fed babies, and when they do get ill it tends to be minor and short-lasting.

A feverish baby requires suckling more often and may need to return to a pattern of almost continuous suckling such as many babies adopt at the end of the first week of life. The mother should have plenty of fluids and as much rest as she can get and, if possible, help with housework or someone who will take it over completely so that she can give her attention to her baby. This is obviously not always feasible but it may be one of the most important things that can be done to help the baby. A breastfed baby who is ill often loses no weight as a result of the illness, whereas an artificially fed baby almost invariably does.

A baby with a respiratory infection and a blocked nose will need nose drops, which can be obtained on prescription from the doctor. She usually sucks in shortened bursts and rests or fusses between. This means that feeds may take longer. On the other hand if she has a high temperature she may tire quickly and drop off the breast before she has taken much. Be ready to suckle again when she stirs. The baby will use the breast for comfort as well as for obtaining nourishment and this is something valuable the mother can give the baby who is uncomfortable or in pain.

When a breastfed baby has to go into hospital the mother should always be able to go with her if she wishes, and stay day and night. It is reasonable to refuse to allow your baby to be admitted to any hospital which cannot accommodate you, and to go to another hospital which will. If the baby is unable to suck following an operation or in an acute illness breast milk can be expressed and tube-fed to the baby. (See page 80.)

After surgery a baby is specially susceptible to infection and may be in pain, which is increased by any sudden change in milk which produces a different kind of stool to be passed. Breast milk fights bacteria which can cause infection and allows for easy assimilation of nutrients. The comfort of the mother's presence is probably also an important factor in quick recovery. The appearance of a baby in intensive care or after an operation can be a shock to the parents, and tubes and other attachments prove repulsive:

He looked so pathetic with two tubes in his stomach and chest, an IV tube on his wrist, and oxygen and heart machines hooked to him ... His gastrostomy made nursing nerve-wracking for me, and painful for him. When he cried, his stomach muscles would tense up and send gas and excess food up the tube. I worried when it overflowed, and I worried when it was empty, for fear he wasn't getting my milk.[8]

Both the mother and father need to be prepared for such feelings and to have emotional support and accurate and full information during this difficult time. Anxiety can interfere with the let-down reflex and a mother who has been separated from her baby may also be having to cope with the problems resulting from engorgement.

When a baby is linked up to machines and has odd tubes

and bits of sticky tape all over the body it is difficult to cuddle her, and nurses and parents may be reluctant to hold and touch the baby except to adjust the apparatus or change a nappy because they are afraid of dislodging the tubing. It is important to work out ways of giving loving through touch. Once the apparatus is no longer required the baby may have to 'catch up' on handling which she has missed and benefits from extended periods of cuddling.

PREGNANT AGAIN

It is possible to go on feeding through a pregnancy if a woman wants to, and it is not necessary to suddenly stop breastfeeding if she thinks she may be pregnant. Weaning from the breast should always take place over a matter of weeks, cutting out one feed at a time. But she may feel that weaning the older child is not likely to be easy at this stage or that it is not right.

Some women find it a strain to continue breastfeeding when they are pregnant and it is possible that some of the physiological, and perhaps also the emotional, resources which the expectant mother has to bring to her pregnancy may be not so readily available if she continues to breastfeed. In most societies mothers wean when another pregnancy is confirmed, and primate mothers usually reject their offspring when they again become pregnant. So there is no reason to think that it is more 'natural' to continue to breastfeed during a subsequent pregnancy. Some women, however, do get an enormous feeling of satisfaction from doing so and breastfeed both children after the birth of the second. This is a personal decision which the woman should feel free to make according to her life-style and her awareness of her own and her child's needs.

Early on in pregnancy the mother who is still lactating following a previous delivery may find that she gets unusual 'drawing' pains in her breasts and they can become acutely tender to touch, as the glandular changes which occur in the first three months of pregnancy get under way. This can amount to considerable pain. It may be incorrectly diagnosed as 'threatened mastitis'. The discomfort may be relieved by wearing a firm bra with wide shoulder straps or, if there is much breast enlargement, by strapping the breasts with a wide elastic bandage. Cold compresses (chips of ice folded into nappies) may also help. The mother may also discover that some time between the second and fifth month her milk supply starts to tail off, until by about the seventh month only a few drops of fluid can be expressed. If she wishes to wean the toddler this seems to be a good time to do so. In one study of 600 American mothers who became pregnant while breastfeeding it was also found that a large percentage of these women experienced irritation with the child they were still breastfeeding.[9]

If a woman does decide to go on breastfeeding right through a subsequent pregnancy she can rest assured that after the initial physiological adjustments of early pregnancy and a reduction of supply in middle and late pregnancy breastfeeding will continue without problems, but it is important to see that her diet is adequate to support both the pregnancy and lactation.

Colostrum will be present in the breasts in the last weeks of pregnancy and following delivery, just as it is with mothers who are not already lactating. This will change to transitional and then to mature milk within a matter of days.

When the older child sees the baby at the breast she will probably want to suckle again and can be cuddled in one's arms at the same time or following the baby's feed, though this should be considered mainly comfort suckling and plays no part in the nutrition of the older child. Suckling two children simultaneously ensures that the mother has periods with the older child when they can both settle down for a quiet time together, so clearing a space for the important short rests that are an integral part of a well-run pregnancy.

12. Everybody else is coping: why can't I?

It is almost an occupational description of mothers that they seek to excel and compete with each other about the development, skills and qualities of their children. When you have your first baby you may have yet to learn the reality of this and that although other mothers may be your best friends they can also lead you to doubt your own capacities and even your right to be a mother.

In the past women used to compete about babies' weight gains but now that the emphasis is on the dangers of rearing babies as if they were pigs being fattened, this has largely shifted, at least among the middle classes, to competition about motor development and intelligence. One of the first races which the new mother feels she is running with her acquaintances who also have new babies is to see who can have the baby who sleeps through the night in advance of the others. Be warned; this will almost certainly be a bottle-fed baby, because since they have a food which is intended for rearing calves who grow a good deal faster than human babies, they are more readily filled up and can go longer between feeds.

The old idea that 'good' babies sleep through the night and that 'naughty' ones wake two or three times dies hard. Your baby is being neither good nor bad if she wakes in the night; she wakes because she needs you, whether this is for food or comfort, or both. You can gradually train her to see that this is not a great social occasion, however bouncing and ready to go she is, by being naturally sleep-sodden and rather uncommunicative yourself and by keeping the room dimly lit and stimulus at a minimum; you can thus emphasize the social difference between the night and the day. But you cannot force a baby to sleep when it does not want to or is not ready.

There are inherent differences between babies in the amount of sleep they need and how long they can comfortably go between feeds. When you come to think of it, these differences also apply to adults. There are statistical averages but, as with all averages, a great many people will be either side of the average figure by a substantial margin. With any average it is 'normal' for just about half the people to be above and half below it. Pretty well half the population is below average height, for instance. It is as well to keep this fact in mind when you talk about your baby's development, compare her progress with any other baby's, or relate it to what is described as normal development in a book. It is knowledge easily forgotten, especially when you begin to get anxious about the 'milestones' she should be reaching. If you are in any doubt about your baby's development or have an uneasy feeling that all is not well, go to the doctor, who will not be emotionally involved in the same way, and he or she will either immediately put your mind at rest or suggest a paediatrician or other expert who can advise you. If your GP cannot help, you can ask to be referred to a paediatrician. Paediatricians do not just study babies; they know a good deal about mothers too and will treat you as an interacting unit, a partnership. They will help you with your worries as well as discovering about the baby's health.

A child's development does not take place in a smooth progression, but in leaps and starts. Just when you think your child is *never* going to drop a 4 a.m. feed, or smile, or sit up, it happens. The same is true of all maturational processes, whether physical or mental. Anna Freud[1] speaks of an 'alternation between progression or regression' as perfectly normal: 'On the whole it is safe to insist that children of all ages should be permitted at times to function below the level of their potentialities without being automatically labelled as "backward" ...' In fact, a regressive phase often heralds a great leap forward.

You will find that other mothers have babies who take a far shorter time to feed than yours, and that while you still have a baby plugged on hard after forty minutes or so, another woman has one who gulped everything down in seven minutes flat and then fell asleep or lay happily cooing. Here again, bottle-fed babies, especially those who have large holes in the teat, are more likely to get adequate nutrition in a short time and can usually beat breastfed babies hollow when it comes to speed at feeding. You have to decide whether that is your aim.

A lot more is going on between the two of you when your baby is at the breast than goes on between the baby and the caretaker, whether mother or somebody else, when a baby is feeding from a bottle, if only because the baby is physically much closer to you and in flesh-to-flesh contact. Communication is altogether more intimate. If you hate it, or are fretting at having to spend so long with a baby who seems like a parasite attached to your breast, negative feelings about what is happening are communicated to the baby too, through muscle tensions, heartbeat, even perhaps the more subtle galvanic skin response and your smell. If you can settle back and accept it, enjoying this unique relationship while you have it, in spite of the unmade bed, the dishes waiting to be washed, and the nappies not yet dried, you communicate positive feelings and provide the baby with the ultimate luxury of *being enjoyed*. Only you know whether this is possible, and nobody else is entitled to judge your decision about breast or bottle feeding under the circumstances, because nobody else can really know how you *feel* when you are giving breast or bottle. These feelings are important, just as important as the baby's weight.

You may also discover that while your baby is being suckled about every two or three hours other mothers have babies who allow them to plan their own lives with regularity and know that they will be soundly sleeping three and a half hours after the last feed. It can seem very unfair. If you had only three hours a day to call your own, organizing the housework and getting yourself washed and dressed, *and* brushing your hair and putting on makeup and getting out to the shops would be easy. As it is, you barely have time even to go to the lavatory. This is where your partner comes in, whether it is your husband or someone else who can help you out through the difficult early days, and everybody needs *some-*

body, whether it is another woman, a teenager who comes in after school, a living-in or daily help (one hour a day is better than five hours one day a week). In simpler societies women always had other women in the extended family to whom to turn and nobody was left trying to cope in isolation.

Arrange to do some of the chores together and for your husband to take over some entirely, even if he thinks these are ones he is not very good at. It will not work if you have to *ask* him all the time. If the baby fusses through the evening as so many babies do, it may be the best time for you to recover in a hot bath while he cares for her for a while. Sipping a drink in the bath, while he has his with the baby, will allow you to recover and to turn into a human being again. Since most babies take time to sleep earlier in the day, do not leave preparation of the evening meal until near the hour you want to have it. Get it over and done with, as far as you can, at whichever part of the day the baby is easiest, so that either of you can do the finishing touches just before you eat. Most mothers find that the evening is the worst time of all and that a baby who could seem adorable at midday becomes unbearable just when they are at their most tired. It is possible that the mother's weariness and the baby's crying are interconnected, and anything which treats the mother's exhaustion may go a good way to relieving the baby's crying in the long run.

Anyone who has never lived through this period of early parenting or who looks back on it from the perspective of years does not really know what the new mother is experiencing. With imagination or an accurate memory they may have some idea, but most older women who give advice, including affectionate mothers and mothers-in-law who want the best for you and your baby, do not remember with any precision what it felt like to be a new mother, and the daily doubts and fears which may beset you. They may be genuinely appalled at the muddle you are living in and a man's mother may worry that he is not being fed well because of this, or that you are neglecting to look after him as *she* looked after him. (I hope you are. He is grown-up now.)

The role of mother is denigrated in our society to such an

extent that many mothers seem to feel the need to excel in each mothering task and to prove that it is important. This concentration of effort on each task, as if one wins or loses according to whether one breastfeeds successfully for nine months, or a year, or eighteen months or whatever, or the baby is into a regular sleeping pattern by six weeks on the dot, or that it never goes down with a cold, or has a sticky eye or a skin rash, *because you are such a good mother*, probably lies at the bottom of women's criticism of other women as mothers and the very harsh judgements that mothers are liable to make about each other.

Once you can solve the problem of competitiveness between mothers and speak honestly to your friends, it helps to have a support group of other new mothers, since almost inevitably most of them will be experiencing the same emotions that you are too. The sad thing is that each isolated woman thinks she is the *only* one to feel this way; that her failure is uniquely hers. But however informal a support group it needs some organizing, and someone has to work up the energy to communicate between its members. Many mothers discover that the group which formed in their antenatal class continues informally afterwards; if it was a couples' class this is all the better. Some of the men in my own antenatal classes help with keeping the group running afterwards, and the couples meet regularly in each other's homes, plan picnics together and babysit for each other sometimes, while the women keep in touch on the phone and meet for coffee during the day. It is sad when an antenatal class prepares women for labour as if they were all sitting an exam, and then abandons them at the time when they most need to share their experiences with others they can trust and who are in a similar situation.

But of course it is not only a question of what others say and think about you, but your own self-image. *None* of us can live up to how we want to be as mothers. Some put a bold front on it but in a culture where mothering has to be a conscious, learned activity and yet one for which there is very inadequate preparation during girlhood and adolescence, self-doubt, a sense of inferiority, anxiety about the outcome of one's actions, are all integral to being a mother. In *The Mother Person*[2] Virginia Barber and Merrill Maguire Skaggs advise:

Many mothers' crises occur on the eighteenth conflict, after we've handled the morning's first seventeen remarkably well. But in our revulsion against our handling of the eighteenth, we forget how well we managed what preceded it. One solution of sorts was supplied by an academic: 'I'm going to start giving myself some As every day. I'm going to grade myself in small periods of time, and I'm not going to remind myself of my overall average. I'm going to say, "Boy, was I splendid between three and three-thirty!" '

Look at any day and you will discover short periods of time when you really did rather well. Those are the ones to remember and to build on.

PROBLEM SOLVING: FINDING YOUR OWN PATTERN

You might start by asking yourself the following questions . . .

Is there anything I like about breastfeeding? If so, what?

Is there anything the baby likes about breastfeeding. If so, what?

Is there anything I dislike about breastfeeding. If so, what?

Is there anything the baby dislikes about breastfeeding? If so, what?

Breastfeeding should be a pleasure for you and the baby.

Quite apart from anything that other people tell you to do, how can you maximize the first two and minimize the second two? This can be the basis of discovering satisfying inter-action for two unique and special individuals, the mother and her baby.

If you have tried many different techniques advised by other people, think through the methods you have found did not work for you. You can probably make quite a collection. Having recollected them, discard them and get them off your mind. It is surprising how often mothers store advice which they have found from experience was useless but which still hangs about and burdens them with the feeling that they ought to try it once more and see if it works now. That way leads to terrible muddle.

Think of specific instances in which feeds were satisfying for you and the baby and you feel you did the right thing. Can you describe in detail exactly what happened? Think it through as if you were a novelist recording minutely every glance, every touch, everything that was said, every thought you had. You might try writing it down.

Now think of a feed that went badly, or a space between feeds that was chaotic, or both if you can, and describe that in just the same detail. It may help to write that down too.

At this point compare the two and note the differences. You will probably find all sorts of clues. It can help to talk it through with your husband too, and he may interpret the 'evidence' rather differently.

How can you recreate the conditions, emotional and physical, for you as well as for the baby, when the feed went well? And is there any way you can plan to avoid the situation when things went badly?

If you have answers to these questions you are learning a good deal about the interaction between you and your baby. This is all your own work. No one is telling you what you ought to do. You are making your personal choices based on your own experience.

'Every day is chaotic ... The baby cries all the time ... I don't know whether it is night or day ... I never have time to do anything else ... We can't go on like this.'

Some people can accept chaos more readily than others and are not worried about it. Either the woman or her husband or both may be the kind of person who gets very anxious when they cannot plan ahead or live in orderly surroundings. Meals on time are an important part of some men's lives. Cleaning up the kitchen and getting the beds made may seem an almost superhuman task to fit in, but one you may feel you simply must do and feel miserable about if you can-

not. Or you may have a commitment to work outside the
home which is looming over you, or free-lance work at home,
or a thesis or report to be written. Babies turn this orderly
sequence of events topsy-turvy. Even more important, some
women never seem to be able to get any time to rest or 'be
themselves' when they have a new baby; they are serving the
baby's needs non-stop. Although twenty-four-hour concern
with the baby's needs can be exciting and fascinating in the
first six to eight weeks, and seems to come quite spontaneously to many women, to carry on in that intense state of
concentration for much longer than that proves very exhausting. If you want to get some shape into your day and work
out when you can do other things and begin to find yourself,
not only as a mother, you may like to make a plan of the
baby's general behaviour. It is much better to do this than
to try to *superimpose* a schedule on the baby.

Use the squared pages at the back of this book. There is
one page for each twelve hours and the six pages will allow
you to record what happened over a three-day period. Each
square corresponds to thirty minutes. You will need symbols
corresponding to different kinds of behaviour in the baby.
Select the dominant behaviour for each half-hour period,

e.g. awake and contented

fussing (or crying)

sucking

sleeping

When you have worked through the three days like this you
will probably be able to get some idea of an emerging pattern, and see where you have spaces and can have a rest or
get on with something else. Your baby may change, so do
not think of this as static, but it will enable you to introduce
a flexible routine into your day if you wish.

13. Breastfeeding in a polluted world

Although breastfeeding is the most natural and wholesome way that a woman can feed her baby, she is not immune from the chemicals which pollute our urban-industrial environment, particularly in the form of pesticides which are used on food crops, and these chemicals may go through her blood stream into her milk. It has been discovered, for example, that DDT passes into breast milk, as it is now present in the milk of all mammals. A study of 1,400 breastfeeding women done in 1976 by the Human Effects Monitoring Branch of the United States Environmental Protection Agency, came to the startling conclusion that breast milk was widely contaminated with pollutants, some of which are known to cause cancer in animals, although no untoward effects of DDT have been observed in babies.[1] Some women have become deeply concerned about this and have even decided that bottle feeding may be safer.

Further research in the United States,[2] however, indicates that a vegetarian diet reduces the amount of DDT in breast milk and that even when the mother is not on a completely vegetarian diet (she may eat fish about once a week, for example) the level is only one third to one half of that found in women eating more conventional diets. The United States Environmental Defence Fund now advises breastfeeding mothers to cut down or cut out meat.

A woman does not, of course, have to eat meat or have any animal products at all if she does not wish to, in order to produce milk. Cows and goats are vegetarians!

There are other pollutants which constitute more of a problem. These are the polychlorinated biphenyls, used in the manufacture of electronics, for example, for several decades. They are called PCBs for short. These potentially toxic compounds have contaminated soil, water, air and food. There is no hard evidence which suggests that it is dangerous to breastfeed, however, because the effect on the baby is not known. These chemicals are probably absorbed by the breastfeeding woman in air and drinking water and perhaps through some household products as well as in food, since the level of PCBs in the milk of vegetarian mothers is not very different from that of non-vegetarian mothers. Research continues, and so far suggests that women who want to give their babies the best chance of a healthy life may have to be prepared to alter their life-styles once we learn exactly what are the greatest dangers in a contaminated world. The chief dietary source of PCBs, for example, is freshwater fish, but in the USA fish marketed commercially must be within the FDA's guidelines for PCBs, although fish caught privately are not monitored in this way. Polybrominated biphenyl (PBB) is another contaminant, closely related to PCB, which was accidentally introduced into the Michigan food supply in 1973 and women on quarantined farms were advised not to breastfeed. Fortunately this was an isolated incident and it looks as if care will now be taken to limit the toxic substances used in industry which can enter our food. But this ought to be a matter for continuing public concern and consumer awareness.

These industrial pollutants are often stored in body fat and in the fat of animals which are eaten. It may be advisable, therefore, to cut down on fats, and some authorities recommend choosing low-fat dairy products such as skim milk, yoghurt and buttermilk, and avoiding sprays and chemicals as far as possible in the home.

Radioactive strontium 90 is also present in breast milk, but there is five times more in cow's milk, so this is one good reason for breastfeeding.[3] As bottle-fed babies get older the strontium body content goes up, whereas that of breastfed babies falls. Breastfeeding helps to protect the baby against damage from radiation.[4]

Lead is also present in breast milk, but here again, at lower levels than in cow's milk and that found in certain brands of fruit juice in lead cans.[5]

There is a kind of jaundice called pregnanediol jaundice which tends to become more marked in the breastfed baby.

There is probably a toxic-environmental cause, and one likely explanation is the association between induction of labour with oxytocin and increased rates of neonatal jaundice.[6] There is no risk of brain damage from this type of jaundice, but paediatricians sometimes advise discontinuing breastfeeding for forty-eight hours so that the bilirubin level can drop, after which breastfeeding can be continued.

CANCER

There have been claims that breastfeeding is a contributory cause of breast cancer, and other claims that it prevents it. It has been known for some time that women who have not borne children are more likely to get breast cancer than those who have. Recent research suggests that breastfeeding protects against cancer which develops after the menopause. No one knows why this is, but it may be that the flow of milk clears the breast tissues of some chemicals which otherwise tend to accumulate and to cause cancerous changes in later life, or that milk produces a protective substance in the breast.

A fishing community living on boats in the delta of the Pearl River, Hongkong, always breastfeed their babies from one breast only, the right one, because their dress traditionally opens this side. A study of the relation between breastfeeding and cancer in these women, done by doctors at the Queen Mary Hospital, Hong Kong, and the Queen Elizabeth Hospital, Kowloon,[7] revealed that twenty-seven out of thirty-four women over fifty-five had breast cancer in the breast which they had not used for feeding. So the claim that breastfeeding reduces the chances of the mother having cancer is valid at least so far as breast cancer developing in later life is concerned.

There has also been anxiety that virus particles discovered in breast milk of mothers whose close relatives have had breast cancer might contribute to the later development of cancer in their babies. It has been suggested that these women should avoid breastfeeding baby girls, even though they are themselves healthy. Workers at the United States

National Cancer Institute[8] have studied this matter and point out that if cancer of the breast was transmitted through human milk one would expect to find it occurring predominantly in female lines of families, whereas it occurs equally in male and female lines. Moreover, where both mothers and daughters have developed breast cancer this is not related to the incidence of breastfeeding. As breastfeeding has declined in the USA the incidence of breast cancer has gone up; if these particles in human milk were aetiological agents in breast cancer we should expect to find rates declining. We should also expect to find more breast cancer in Third World societies and cultural groups in the West where breastfeeding is the norm, but the opposite is the case. We can conclude, therefore, that breastfeeding daughters, even if one's mother and other relatives had breast cancer, does not contribute to the likelihood of the girls developing cancer in later life.

DRUGS

It is rarely necessary to stop breastfeeding because you are having drug treatment for an illness, but you should always remind the doctor that you are breastfeeding before he prescribes anything. Even though some drugs used in treatment or for diagnostic procedures enter the breast milk in appreciable quantities, there are nearly always alternatives which can be used. On the whole, little is known about the concentration of any drug in breast milk and since it is unethical to do research on nursing mothers and babies, recommendations have to be based on careful observation of babies to see if drugs taken by their mothers are affecting them, bearing in mind that to wean a baby suddenly because the mother has become ill is likely to be psychologically traumatic for both.

Chemicals present in breast milk depend on their lipid-solubility, their binding capacity with protein, and their degree of ionization.[9] Drugs usually have a higher concentration in the mother's blood stream than in her breast milk, but this is affected by the constitution of the milk. Since the fat content of milk is higher in the morning and as each breast empties, drugs which are fat soluble, such as seconal and phenobarbitone, diffuse into the milk more readily as the fat content increases.[10] Colostrum has a low fat content, so these drugs are unlikely to pass to the baby in the first days after delivery.

On the other hand in the first days of life enzyme systems which normally allow a baby to cope with drugs the mother is taking are not yet operating. Rothermel and Faber[11] warn that some sulpha drugs used to treat urinary tract infections pass into breast milk, can cause jaundice and should be avoided. They advise that sulphonamides should not be used until the baby is two months old.

An occasional aspirin, codeine or other analgesic for a headache is unlikely to affect the baby, although if aspirin is taken just before putting the baby to the breast it could have the effect of slowing down the time it takes for the baby's blood to clot. So if you want to take aspirin, do so *after* a feed. Aspirin is sometimes prescribed in large quantities for rheumatoid arthritis and in this case the effect on the baby should be very carefully watched.

Some anticoagulants are contraindicated for breastfeeding mothers, but others, oral Warfarin or Heparin by injection,[12] are available which are present only in small quantities in the milk and appear to have no effect on the baby.

Some laxatives taken by the mother can give the baby diarrhoea, though cathartics such as milk of magnesia or methyl cellulose and faecal softeners (dioctyl sodium sulphate) are usually all right, and some women can take senna, cascara, aloin and rhubarb-based preparations without causing problems in the baby. But if you take any laxatives be on the look out for diarrhoea in the baby. It is better to change your diet. (See Chapter 14.)

Sleping pills make the baby sleepy too, and some babies come out in a rash when their mothers are taking barbiturates, but if you desperately need sleep for the odd night or two it is a question of balancing the risks and carefully observing any effect on the baby. If you have had barbiturates you may need someone to wake you when the baby wakes for a night feed and to stay awake until the feed is over and the baby settled down again.

Mood-changing drugs prescribed for anxiety and depression can also affect the baby. Valium (diazepam) has sometimes been found to cause lethargy and loss of weight in the baby. Largactil (chlorpromazine) may lead to jaundice. Tofranil, Parnate and Ritalin appear to have no effect in normal doses. If you are keen to breastfeed and are depressed or anxious, weaning the baby *may* make you feel even worse because doing so seems to provide proof that you cannot cope and are no good as a mother. It is usually much more helpful for someone to give emotional support.

Tranquillizers may also create further problems for the mother. Valium, for example, may 'invoke languor which makes the bare necessities of housework, child care and mothering an overwhelming task'.[13] Even though tranquillizers are often freely prescribed by general practitioners for new mothers who suffer from mild depression or who are in a state of constant anxiety about the baby and their ability to mother adequately, research by Margaret Lynch in Oxford has shown that they can be dangerous because they lower the normal controls in behaviour. Women who batter their babies have often sought help from their general practitioners, who have prescribed tranquillizers. Under the influence of these tranquillizing drugs they more readily act on impulse and physically abuse their babies.

Although most oral antibiotics can safely be taken, some babies develop an allergy to penicillin. On others it has no adverse effect. It is theoretically possible that tetracycline may colour the teeth yellow, since it may have this effect when taken by the mother during pregnancy, but since it is bound to calcium it may not be absorbed.[14] Erythromycin, one of the basic antibiotics, is probably all right before the mature milk is being produced, since it needs an acidic medium for diffusion, and colostrum is alkaline. Whole milk comes in during about the third week after birth, and erythromycin then reaches six times the concentration in breast milk that it has in the mother's blood stream.

Women who suffer from migraine should not take ergot

preparations. They may cause vomiting and diarrhoea, a weak pulse and unstable blood pressure in the baby.

Steroids may gradually build up in the baby, and any effects should be monitored if they are taken over a prolonged period. A short course of about a week is unlikely to cause trouble. Although some doctors believe that diuretics can be used with extreme caution, the USA Federal Drugs Administration has stated that they should not be prescribed for nursing mothers.[15]

Antihistamines seem to be tolerated except that they make the baby drowsy.

Epinephrine, a bronchial dilator, is destroyed in the baby's gastro-intestinal tract and has no effect.

Similarly, insulin taken by the diabetic mother is destroyed in the baby's digestive tract and causes no harm, but if any oral antidiabetic agents are prescribed their effect should be very carefully watched.

Atropine lowers milk production and should not be taken.

Cardiac drugs, such as digitalis, are sometimes given to babies and little is know about the blood-plasma ratio of these substances when they are taken by the breastfeeding mother. If they are prescribed their effect should be carefully monitored.

Oral contraceptives, which are very widely prescribed, are not without risk, mainly because they often reduce the milk flow. So if you feel that the pill is the best contraceptive for you, it is best left till the milk supply is well established. Use a mechanical contraceptive till then. Some authorities advise waiting until the baby is six months old before going on the pill. But a great many mothers have breastfed successfully while taking the contraceptive pill. Watch for possible effects on milk production and be ready to feed more frequently if this is your preferred method of contraception.

If a woman needs to have diagnostic radioactive iodine she should not breastfeed for twenty-four to forty-eight hours following the test dose, and some authorities believe that she should not even have contact with her baby during this time. La Leche recommends that the mother should keep away from the baby for only six hours.[16]

You can safely be vaccinated yourself while breastfeeding, including smallpox, typhoid typhus, rabies, tetanus and cholera vaccines.

Smoking contaminates breast milk with nicotine, though in practice the worst effect seems to be the smoke which is inhaled by the baby, especially in an allergic or nicotine-sensitive baby.[17] So cut out, or, if this is impossible, cut down, on cigarettes. We do not know for certain the effects of heavy smoking on the baby, except that in pregnancy it tends to stunt foetal growth, and large quantities of nicotine may reduce the milk supply. On the other hand, if sitting down for a quiet cigarette makes all the difference to you it is better to do this than to drag on longing for one.

Heavy indulgence in alcohol also reduces the milk supply, but moderate use may actually help you breastfeed better by encouraging the let-down reflex and helping relaxation. The baby of an alcoholic mother may be born already addicted and undergo severe alcohol withdrawal symptoms following delivery.

The baby of a mother addicted to heroin or other hallucinogens also suffers withdrawal symptoms just as if it had itself been addicted. In a large Brooklyn hospital I have seen tiny newborns twitching and jerking as they were taken off the heroin they had been receiving from their mothers' blood streams. Their cribs were padded so they did not rub off skin. These babies have a high-pitched cry, vomit frequently and tend to have a highly uncoordinated sucking reflex so that feeding is difficult. Heroin is secreted in breast milk, and the mother who is addicted should not breastfeed.

Little is known about the effects of cannabis. In one rural commune where mothers customarily breastfeed and also smoke 'grass' the children appear healthy. But these commune members live an outdoor life, are not exposed to other chemical pollutants and are strict vegetarians. It may be that if a breastfeeding mother living under inferior environmental conditions smokes cannabis regularly her baby would be adversely affected. The truth is that we just do not know, and for this reason *all* drugs should be taken with caution, bearing in mind that it may not be the presence or absence of one pollutant which is the decisive factor, but the interaction of varied toxic substances in the mother's environment and personal life-style.

While breastfeeding it is necessary to weigh up the risks to mother and baby of taking or not taking a particular drug. A short course of antibiotics may be needed, for example, and may be well worth any possible side-effects on the baby. The dosage and the duration of time during which drugs are taken obviously must influence the decision. If a very toxic drug must be taken over a short period you will probably decide not to continue breastfeeding during that time. But there is no need to wean the baby. Express the breast milk, using an electric pump for preference (the Egnell pump can be hired through the National Childbirth Trust). The Trust may be able to help you, through its Breastfeeding Promotion Group, by putting you in touch with nursing mothers willing to provide your baby with breast milk during this period. This milk is usually collected over a period of twenty-four hours, stored in the fridge, and then provided bottled.

14. The food you eat

Good breastfeeding depends on the mother having good nutrition. As with everything else, if she looks after herself, she can then look after the baby. If she neglects herself and thinks it does not matter, or goes on to a stringent diet because she wants to get her figure back quickly, breastfeeding will suffer and she will soon feel weary and run-down. The first consequence of under-nutrition may well be emotional. Fatigue is the primary ingredient of depression. The woman, her baby and her marriage, may suffer.

Computer programmers say 'Garbage in; garbage out!' Not a bad motto for the breastfeeding mother! But it is not strictly true, and remarkable what a woman on an inadequate diet can get away with. Her baby flourishes, but she herself is depleted of nutritional reserves. So in another sense the saying is accurate, because some constituents of a good diet, such as vitamin C, need to be obtained every day by the mother and are then passed on in her milk to the baby. The vitamin C content of human milk is entirely dependant on the mother's daily intake. If she is getting oranges, grapefruit, satsumas and tomato or citrus juice, for example, each day, she does not need to give the baby juice until the baby shows an interest in what she is drinking and it is fun to share some of it.

For any woman who is on a poorly balanced or inadequate diet, breastfeeding provides a tremendous nutritional stress, so it is worth reviewing what you are eating and checking to see that you are getting optimum nutrition in terms not only of calories but of protein, vitamins and minerals. A breast-feeding woman does not need to stuff herself, weigh out foods or take pills or other dietary supplements, and there is certainly no need to be faced with enormous food bills. But it is important to get the 'feel' of a good diet and make sure that she does not go without the essential constituents of a well-balanced diet.

A baby usually takes about 2½oz (70g) of breast milk per pound (450g) of his own body weight every day. The mother needs to cater for this in her own diet; she may require approximately 500 more calories, and take this amount extra *without gaining weight*.

Underfed women on a diet poor in protein produce more milk if their protein intake is increased.[1] If the diet is inadequate in protein increasing the protein content can soon produce more milk, although it will not increase its protein content.

A breastfeeding woman does not need to drink milk to produce milk, and it is possible to breastfeed successfully without drinking any milk at all. But she requires a good supply of other protein foods; meat, fish, cheese, eggs, yoghurt, butter or margarine are all first-class proteins. Soya beans are also a first-class protein in that they contain the essential amino acids and are as high in protein as meat. If a woman does not eat animal products she can get protein from soya beans and sprouts, wheat germ, brewer's yeast, nuts and seeds (e.g. sunflower, sesame and pumpkin), whole grain (wheat, oats, rye, rice, wholewheat pasta), dried beans of all kinds, peas and lentils. Few vegetables have a protein content; avocado is one of them. (Avocado is superb cut in chunks and added before the final minute of cooking to scrambled eggs.)

Good books to help you if you prefer a diet without animal products are: *Whole Earth Cookbook*, by Sharon Cadwallader and Judi Ohr, Penguin Books, 1973; *Recipes for a Small Planet*, by Ellen Buchman Ewald, New York, Ballantine, 1973; *Vegetarian Gourmet Cookery*, by Alan Hooker, London, Pitman, 1976; *The Vegetarian Epicure*, by Anna Thomas, Penguin Books, 1974; and *Wings of Life*, by Julie Jordan, New York, The Crossing Press, 1976.

There is no need to make a cult of feeding and it will not help to spend time worrying about balancing your diet, but it is worth getting into good *habits* of diet, if possible well in advance of the birth of your baby. Make sure that you are not eating 'junk' foods, but that everything you and your family consume is of the best quality. When you get the chance to put your feet up in pregnancy or when you are feeding the baby take time to learn about food values and good nutrition, plan meals and write out your shopping list.

If you make your own whole grain bread, to which you can add a handful of soya flour and extra wheat germ (inside the loaf, not on top, as the extreme heat involved in baking the crust destroys some of the value of the germ) you will probably find that an afternoon rest allows enough time for the dough to rise with the trays and tins slipped inside 'swing-bin' plastic bags, and that the length of a breastfeed is about right for proving the finished loaves and rolls. Make three pounds or a couple of kilos of bread at one time and you can freeze what you do not need immediately.

When a woman is going to be in the house anyway with a new baby it is a good time to try out bread recipes and do things she may not have time to do when facing a busy day in the office. Although a lot of time will be taken up with the baby, bread-making is one of the tasks that can easily be fitted in around feeds and babycare. It does a good deal for the new mother's morale to look back on the baby-oriented day when her offspring is having an evening 'cry-in' and think, 'Well, the day was taken up with the baby and maybe I'm not doing too well yet, but I did make some gorgeous bread as well!'

If you like cheese it is a good idea to keep a wide selection of different cheeses in a large plastic container with a firmly fitting lid in the bottom of the fridge. Wrap each one in cling-film so that the flavours do not mingle and you can see what it is. That way, with fresh bread and some beer or wine and a fruit basket, you have a meal however time-consuming the baby has been. It may not be the correct way to keep cheese, but a round of Brie will last four weeks or so under these conditions and a Stilton, with its lid carefully replaced and the whole wrapped in foil, will last for longer still. Take all cheeses out of the fridge an hour or so before the meal so that they can return to room temperature. Any bits of hard cheese can be used up by making potted cheese (although to start with try only one type of cheese at a time); mix 8oz (200g) cheese with approximately 3oz (75g) butter, herbs, finely chopped garlic if you like it, or caraway seeds for a change, salt, pepper, ale or red or white wine, port or madeira, brandy or calvados, till it forms a paste. Put in a pot; cover with foil and keep in the fridge.

It is very dull to have to think constantly about the constituents of diet in terms of proportions of vitamins and so on. Although it is a good idea to look at your diet and see how you can improve it, it is a pity to pass every day concerned with such matters when there is good food to be eaten and *enjoyed*. This is why I believe it is better to work out a well-balanced and optimally nutritious diet for lactation during your quiet times and think through how you could ring the changes on it, and then put it to the back of your mind while you experiment with variations on the main themes and produce dishes you and your family like eating.

Just as it is not only what you feed your baby on but also the atmosphere in which you feed her that is important, so the pleasure with which meals are eaten, and relaxing while having them, is just as important as consuming carefully balanced nutrients. A candle on the table at an evening meal and a romantic atmosphere, or a bunch of primroses at breakfast may do more for the digestion and health of body and mind than a bottle of multi-vitamin pills or dried seaweed in the soup.

So take this information lightheartedly and avoid making a heavy chore of getting the correct nutrients. A woman who is not overweight and who has an active life normally needs about 2,000 calories a day during her childbearing years to be at the peak of health and vitality. When she is pregnant she benefits from having another 300 calories and when she is breastfeeding about another 200 on top of that; this means that she is then having some 500 or 600 extra calories. Anything else she takes will be stored in fat and may be difficult to lose when she stops lactating. When she is not pregnant or lactating, 1½oz (41g) of protein are sufficient, but when pregnant her protein requirements rise to 2oz (61g) and when lactating to 2¼oz (65g). Some of the most important vitamin and mineral needs are as follows:

> Iron – from 14 mg a day to 15 in both pregnancy and lactation. Vitamin C – from 30 mg normally to 50 mg in pregnancy and 60 mg during lactation.
> International units of Vitamin D – 100 in the non-pregnant state; this needs to be doubled for pregnancy and lactation.
> 700 mg of calcium and phosphorus are normally sufficient, but nearly double that is required during pregnancy and lactation – 1,200 mg is then the recommended daily intake.
> The intake of B vitamins should be increased, niacin by half as much again.

The Canada Department of Health and Welfare Committee for Revision of the Canadian Dietary Standard has set out all this in the form of a table in its report of 1975:[2]

RECOMMENDED DAILY NUTRIENT INTAKE FOR WOMEN 19–35 YEARS

Nutrient	Normal activity	Pregnancy	Lactation
energy (Kcal)	2,100	2,400	2,600
protein (g)	41	61	65
thiamin (mg)	1·1	1·3	1·5
niacin (NE)	14	16	21
riboflavin (mg)	1·3	1·6	1·9
vitamin C (mg)	30	50	60
vitamin A (RE)	800	900	1,200
vitamin D (IU)	100	200	200
calcium (mg)	700	1,200	1,200
phosphorus (mg)	700	1,200	1,200
iron (mg)	14	15	15

Notice that the requirements while you are breastfeeding are in most cases even greater than when pregnant. What this really means is that when you increase your diet to give the necessary calories items should be chosen which provide these valuable nutrients. Here are some of the foods to choose from to get these:

Vitamin C is not stored in the body, so you need a selection of foods rich in vitamin C every day. Tomatoes, potatoes cooked in their skins (the English have traditionally obtained most of their vitamin C from potatoes!), all citrus fruits, nasturtium leaves (can be put in sandwiches), blackcurrants, strawberries, sprouts, cabbage, swedes, cauliflower, watercress, mustard and cress, red and green peppers, lettuce and other salad vegetables. (It is lost by cooking, so if you are choosing cabbage, for example, as a source of vitamin C, have it as coleslaw.)

Vitamin A. Fish liver oils, liver, egg yolk, butter, margarine, milk, cheese, eggs, carrots, dark green vegetables such as turnip tops, kale, spinach, watercress and parsley, tomatoes, dried fruits.

The B vitamins. Milk, dried milk, organ meats, fish, cod roe, poultry, cheese, yoghurt, brewer's yeast, yeast extract, tea, peanuts and peanut butter, wholemeal ('wheatmeal' is not the same as 'wholemeal' or 'granary' bread which contains the whole of the wheat, including the germ, which is an important source of B vitamins) bread and flour, cereals and pasta, eggs, soya products, sesame seeds (put on bread or in biscuits or buy tahini paste), brazil nuts, oats, peas (fresh and frozen), mushrooms, chicory, green vegetables, Guinness, sunflower seeds, cashew nuts.

Iron. Meat, fish, poultry, brewer's yeast, pumpkin seeds, whole grains, wheat germ, porridge oats, parsley (a couple of bunches of chopped parsley make a good soup when added to a thin béchamel sauce with finely chopped onion and grated cheese), watercress and other leafy green vegetables, eggs, prunes, raisins, sultanas, dried apricots and other dried fruits, baked beans, soya beans and flour, lentils, yeast and yeast products (e.g. Marmite, Yeastrel), black molasses (a little goes a long way, but it is good in a dark ginger and spice cake and also to bring out the full flavour of a sweet curry sauce), cocoa, chocolate, bananas, nuts, potatoes, sunflower seeds. (Spinach and rhubarb reduce the amount of iron that can be absorbed from food.)

Calcium. Milk, cheese (especially Parmesan), eggs, almonds, brazil nuts, sesame seeds, cabbage, broccoli, water-

cress, potatoes, soya products, oats and oatmeal, dried apricots.

Phosphorus. Brewer's yeast, wheat germ, pumpkin seeds,
sunflower seeds, sesame seeds (these five foods can usually
be bought at health food stores in different appetizing forms),
brazil nuts, cocoa, Parmesan cheese.

If you want to find out more about food values *Diet for a
Small Planet*[3] is a good book to read.

Vitamin B_{12} is the vitamin a vegetarian has to be certain of
getting. Lacto-vegetarians can obtain enough, but Vegans
and those on macro-biotic diets may not have sufficient unless they take tablets of B_{12}, a non-animal product which is
synthesized from mould. Small amounts of B_{12} are obtained
from yeast, wheatgerm and soya beans, but the pregnant and
nursing mother needs more than she could ever get even from
a diet rich in these foods. One result of dietary deficiency in
this vitamin is anaemia. Symptoms are tiredness – including
waking up tired – headaches, depression, a general feeling of
joylessness and of not being able to cope, and a sense of
'What's the point of it all? I don't know what's wrong with
me, but I don't feel right.' This is so often the syndrome of
malaise characteristic of chronic postnatal depression that if
you are not enjoying being a mother it is worth examining
your diet carefully to make certain that you are getting
enough iron, vitamin B_{12} and protein, which the vitamin
must have if it is to be released so that your body can use it.
Even if you are not a vegetarian it is wise to check that
you are getting sufficient of the B vitamins, especially vitamin
B_{12}.

You may like to keep a polythene bag of mixed nuts and
dried fruits for when you are getting overwrought or have no
time for a meal. This same mixture can also be added to raw
oats and wheatflakes to make a muesli mixture with fresh
grated apple, milk and honey or soft brown sugar.

If you select a mixed salad for one meal of the day you
can be sure about your vitamin C intake. But do not make do
with the ordinary tossed salad with a rather dull lettuce and
little bits of nondescript vegetables. Experiment with different combinations on a large flat meat plate or trencher

and keep a selection of home-made dressings in a cool place. Going by colour is a good guide: you need something green, something white or yellow and something orange or red as a basic minimum. Mix fruits and vegetables if your partner does not object to his salad being half the dessert!

Put your imagination into the first course and serve fruit for pudding or whip up a quick syllabub/mousse in an electric mixer with 8 oz (250g) of cream, half a glass of sweet wine, 1 teaspoon lemon juice and a little icing sugar, or the same amount of cream with a few teaspoons of brandy, rum, advocaat or a couple of tablespoons of ginger marmalade, melted cooled dark chocolate or sweetened fruit purée (raspberry, strawberry or blackcurrant are good). Chill well in little pots.

A thick 'everything goes' soup can be a meal in itself with your home-made bread and a good cheese plate, or it can precede a salad. 'Everything goes' soup depends on not wasting anything, on having an electric blender large enough to take the solid ingredients and on having some onions. Sauté onions in oil or butter, add left-over vegetables (you will soon get to know good combinations) and then either thicken with potato, a cornflower roux or a béchamel or white sauce. Add stock, water, milk or a mixture, and herbs (basil is good with tomato and a good many other mixtures) and cook and taste and season till it seems right. If you have no fresh vegetables use a tin of sweet corn; thicken with white sauce and milk, and add plenty of black pepper, salt and nutmeg. Or you can top an onion soup with cheese-laden thin barques of French bread and brown under the grill. You can use a tin of chestnut purée (unsweetened) or some ground roasted peanuts instead of vegetables, or a tin of tomato purée. It is well worth having a good soup recipe book against which to test your inspirations rather than to follow meticulously. Good ones are in Arabella Boxer's *Garden Cook Book*, Sphere, 1977, and Rose Elliot's *Not Just a Load of Old Lentils*, Fontana, 1976. (I am a vegetarian and so may be overlooking good recipe books which specialize in meat cookery.)

The mother of the 'colicky' baby can quickly get to the end of her tether and find that she has no time to eat. You owe it to yourself and your baby to keep up your strength. The baby who fusses all evening is often sleeping at breakfast time, so settle for a good breakfast, even if this is not your usual style of living. If you like, take it back to bed on a tray and imagine you are in a luxury hotel, or settle on getting it brought to you by someone who loves you! It should include a main protein dish and fruit or juice. An enriched milk-shake (a glass of milk with an ice cube, with a banana or some blackcurrant, strawberry or raspberry purée, sweetened to taste and blended till frothy) or an egg flip (for example, 2 eggs, juice of 2 oranges, 1 pint (6dl) very cold milk, a spoonful of runny honey, blended till frothy and kept in the fridge for not longer than twelve hours) may be the answer later on in the day, together with nuts and fruit in a big bowl attractively displayed near your bed or wherever you rest and have the main baby sessions. (Much better than chocolate or toffee under the pillow!) If fruit is expensive think of the electricity or gas you are saving in not cooking, and buy the best-quality fruit you can afford in as wide a variety as you can manage.

FOOD IN HOSPITAL

In a study of the views on breastfeeding held by health visitors and midwives it was found that as many as 31 per cent of the sample believed that fruit and vegetables should be limited or even omitted entirely from the breastfeeding mother's diet![4]

When you are in hospital you may find that someone tells you that you should not eat grapes, for example, which nurses often think cause 'wind' in babies, and later on people may tell you that onions, or curry or garlic, strawberries or any strong-tasting food are bad for your milk. This is not true. One wonders how ever Indian babies could have survived if curry 'contaminated' breast milk or how Mexican babies fare when their mothers eat hot pepper paste. Although hot spicy sauces are not an essential part of your diet, fruit and vegetables are. They are vitally important in the days immediately following delivery for the sake of your own health, since this is often a time when women suffer from constipation.

It is normal not to have a bowel motion for three or four days after childbirth. The bowel was cleared out physiologically by the processes of labour, and you may have had an enema or suppositories to start with as well. It is unlikely that you ate much, if at all, during labour, and your body needs a space of time in which to cope with all the mechanics of digestion and excretion after the momentous physiological impact of the birth. So do not get anxious when nurses regularly ask you if you have 'been' in the first three or four days after the delivery. Drink plenty of fluids; important because after delivery your body is excreting the fluids you have retained in late pregnancy, much of them through the sweat glands in your skin. Hospitals tend to be hot places, and may be deliberately kept so for the sake of the babies. This will increase your fluid loss. Drink as much as you want and even a little more, because in this way you will help your bowels to work when they are ready. Drinking excessively does *not* help produce more breast milk, and may even reduce the supply. You need sufficient liquid, and will probably feel very thirsty, especially when the baby starts to feed, so have a glass of water or some juice or tea ready at your side to sip then. But your own inclinations are as good a guide as any.

Plenty of fresh fruit (apples are especially good) and salads (raw carrot is helpful), with roughage in the form of muesli or bran, really coarse wholemeal bread, honey, rhubarb, and prunes, dates, dried apricots, yoghurt or figs will soon get your bowels working normally. Unfortunately few hospitals provide this kind of diet, and chips, mashed potato, some limp meat in gravy and overcooked 'greens' will do nothing to help you. So it may be a good idea to supplement the hospital diet by getting the kind of food you need brought in. When I was working in Jamaica I discovered that the standard remedy for constipation among Jamaican peasant women was to eat grapefruit regularly, *including* the pithy white part next to the skin. And, although I cannot envisage your husband bringing these in paper bags for you to consume, boiled onions are also very good, and delicious with plenty of black pepper and a pat of butter.

If you are inactive for any length of time you may face more difficulty in getting a normal bowel rhythm. This is one reason why getting moving soon after childbirth is wise, and why even if you are in bed you should practise frequent exercising of the muscles. Simply pulling all your abdominal muscles well in and pressing the small of your back against a firm surface such as the mattress, holding it for a count of five, releasing, and doing it again five times, and repeating this every half hour, will help.

Unfortunately some aperients pass into your breast milk and tend to affect the baby. (See Chapter 13.)

If there *is* any food which your baby's digestion cannot cope with you will know and he will usually develop a rash. These things happen far less often than is commonly thought, but occasionally a baby develops pink blotches after a mother has gorged herself on chocolate, and if you get eczema or asthma you may find that any food to which you have yourself a half-suspected allergy, which in the past you have not taken much notice of, is reacted to by the baby. If a baby has any tendency to react to protein foods and you go on to an all-egg 'slimming' diet, for example, you can tell from his restless behaviour that he is not happy with it. On the whole you can be sure that any food which is good for you is also good for your baby.

Smoking is not a good idea while breastfeeding, as nicotine passes through your milk into the baby, and it may also reduce your milk supply. On the other hand, if you feel that an occasional cigarette is important for you to be able to relax, it may be better for you to be a relaxed smoking mother than a tense non-smoking one. Only you can judge. But if you do smoke, the limit should be two or three a day.

A glass of wine, cider or beer with a meal provides extra fluid and acts as a gentle tranquillizer. A glass of sherry, a Pimm's or a cocktail to sip when you are facing a feed after which you know the baby is unlikely to settle in the evening, can help both you and your husband cope with the situation with greater equanimity! Guinness contains brewer's yeast which, because it is rich in B vitamins, is especially good for breastfeeding mothers. In some hospitals Guinness is provided 'on the house' during the postpartum stay.

If you drink too much alcohol your baby may act slightly drunk. The most usual reaction seems to be for the baby to sleep it off very heavily. Some mothers have said that this happened, for example, after they had been to a wedding and had celebrated with rather too much champagne. You are hardly likely to get into a habit of drinking champagne in this quantity, and probably once in a while does not matter. But do not have a baby sleeping in bed with you if you are aware that you have a level of alcohol which may make you sleep very heavily. Pull the cot up close to the bed instead. If you or your husband feel you need help with a drinking problem, a new baby is a good reason for ringing Alcoholics Anonymous.

15. Communication and relationships

THE BABY SEES

Although mothers may still sometimes be told that their newborn babies 'can't see', in fact they see rather well, though within a limited range. The point of sharpest focus is approximately nine inches away, which is about the distance of a mother's face when she is breastfeeding.[1] Although a mother who is bottle feeding her baby may hold her baby at this distance from her face, she can feed him turned at an angle away from her, and some people, not realizing the importance of being face to face with a baby, do this. In hospitals nurses may even bottle feed babies while they are lying in their cots in a position where there is no chance of nurse and baby looking at each other. It is difficult to breastfeed in anything *other* than the right position.

Objects outside the baby's range of vision are out of focus, although she is aware of light and dark and movement. Within her range a baby can see different contours and planes, and prefers a patterned to a plain surface and complex to simple patterns. But most of all she likes to look at a human face. She is attracted to the shine of eyes, the varied movements of the mouth, and her mother's head coming towards her and turning from side to side and at different angles. And even by two weeks of age a baby prefers her mother's face to a strange woman's face, and may withdraw her gaze and look almost over the stranger's shoulder.[2]

THE BABY HEARS

The newborn can also hear well, responds most readily to the patterned sounds produced by the human voice and prefers high frequency sounds typical of a woman's voice.[3] Adults spontaneously talk to babies in high-pitched voices, and on a tape recording of one of our own baby's births there is a marked difference between the voice my husband used in talking to me and that he adopted as he spoke to the newborn baby and asked, 'What shall we call you, little thing?'

THE BABY RECOGNIZES SMELLS

From early on the baby also knows her mother by smell. Two-day-old babies respond to different odours, such as aniseed or phenyl alcohol, by changes in breathing and heart-rate. Aidan Macfarlane[4] tested two-day-old and six-day-old breast-fed babies and found that at two days babies preferred a breast pad which had been inside their mother's brassière to clean ones. By six days they had already come to prefer their own mother's pad to a strange mother's pad, and this was even more pronounced by ten days. Breast milk alone does not have this effect; the baby is drawn to her mother's smell.

THE BABY LEARNS

From the psychologist's point of view the newborn baby 'is not a passive, featureless organism whose sole objective is to reduce discomfort to a minimum. Rather, he is from birth an active, frequently alert, unique being, capable of sensory discriminations, or learning, and of directing his attention towards those stimuli that are likely to be of greatest significance.'[5]

From the first weeks of life the baby actively searches for stimulus. Daniel Stern makes an analogy between the function of stimulation for the brain and that of food for the body: 'Just as food is needed for the body to grow, stimulation is needed to provide the brain with the "raw materials" required for the maturation of perceptional, cognitive, and sensory motor processes.'[6]

But stimulation, like food, can be of the wrong kind, can come at the wrong time, when the baby is not ready for it, and can be provided in excess. One of the first things that parents learn about their new baby is what stimulus she enjoys, when it is best given and exactly how much works best.

A baby is most ready to enjoy and learn from stimulation when in a quiet, alert state. She is completely awake, attentive to what is happening round her, breathing evenly and with her eyes wide open. It is an immediately recognizable state of *awareness*. A perceptive mother and father pick up a special readiness for stimulation when the baby is like this and talk and interact with her then.

A baby is rarely completely alert when lying on her back,[7] so this is not a good position in which always to put her down. Paediatricians often examine babies and test their responses when they are lying flat. They would probably get very different results in terms of assessing infant behaviour if the babies were well propped up.

THE BABY COMMUNICATES

The baby has a repertoire of sounds and cries which elicit different responses from her parents. Mothers usually know what the cries mean without having to think about it. The more analytical they get, the less they may be able to interpret them. When records of babies crying in hunger, then pain, then boredom or mild irritation were played to mothers and they were asked to say what each cry meant, without thinking too much about their replies, they knew immediately.

John Newson makes the bold statement that 'human babies become human beings because they are treated as if they already were human'.[8] The conversations that parents have with their baby, from birth on, are important not because the baby understands them in a way that adults comprehend the words, but because they prepare her for joining in such conversations later and to be a human and therefore a *social* being. Any baby is at an advantage in learning to become human if she is provided with an environment in which she discovers that her own actions affect other people's behaviour and that she can influence what happens around her. A baby who is not just acted on by those caring for her, but who can interact with them, send them messages, anticipate their responses and make effective *transactions*, is being given the basis for mastering new skills, exploring ideas and entering into satisfying social relationships as she grows up.

So stimulus alone is not enough. It is not a matter of bombarding a baby with colours and sounds, hanging everything one can find round the cot, or producing a vast variety of toys as soon as he can grasp. It is rather a matter of being alert to share with the baby sequences of interaction in which one gives and the other takes, then one takes and the other gives. Simultaneously a foundation is laid for all later communication and the child learns that he is not helpless in the face of life, but can explore, control and master the environment.

Such transactions begin as soon as the baby's eyes are first fixed on the mother's face after delivery and she says something like, 'Look, she's opened her eyes. She's looking at me! Hello, funny one!'

Breastfeeding is not only a matter of getting milk into a baby and filling up its stomach as a car is filled up with petrol. It is also *communication*, giving a unique experience of physical intimacy and skin contact with the mother and interrelationship with her. In breastfeeding the baby is of necessity touched and held close much more than in bottle feeding, the baby's mouth and cheek rest against the mother's flesh and little hands may explore her breast. It is, of course, perfectly possible to hold a baby close against one's body also when bottle feeding, but even if the mother decides that she would like to have the baby's face against her bare breast she is unlikely to choose to do this at every feed. To do this becomes a slightly artificial set 'exercise'. It happens quite naturally and without any conscious deliberation with breastfeeding.

Some women find the sheer repetitiveness of breastfeeding extremely boring and prefer the bottle because then someone else can give the feed. Babies spend a very large part of their lives feeding, and unless the mother can see something more in the process than filling up the baby with milk it is true that the whole procedure can become a tedious duty.

The time at the breast can be a rich experience for the

baby. Much is happening over and above nutritional activity. The very first conversations between mother and baby start with the touch of nipple, mouth, tongue, jaw and cheek; with smell and eye contact. The observant mother quickly becomes aware of changed breathing and sucking rhythms. The baby progresses to more varied and exploratory touch as she discovers the mother's body and to more subtle non-verbal communication, the beginning of sounds and the rudiments of speech.

In the way she holds, touches and speaks to the baby at the breast the mother is presenting the way she sees the world, and is conveying to the baby the message that it is a lovely, safe place or a dangerous and frightening one. The message is communicated through her own muscle tensions, her facial expression, the tone and rhythms of her voice, the readiness with which she responds to and adapts to her baby's signals or perhaps the determination with which she holds it like a rigid package which must be dealt with or the limpness with which she lets it lie on her lap without really being aware of all that is going on.

D. W. Winnicott once suggested that during feeding the baby was gathering stuff for dreaming. The fantasies which become an integral part of the baby's developing psychic life are formed during feeds and in the intervals between suckling. A mother who watches her baby during a satisfying feed sees the child wholly, completely involved in an intense experience, even quivering with passion and delight as she suckles, right down to the feet and toes, and as she is increasingly satiated the eyelids become half closed with what seems to be sensuous experience.

A mother is often overwhelmed by the sheer reality and vitality of the baby in her arms, the almost savage vigour which the baby brings to feeding, and the manner in which it rises to the nipple like a trout snapping a fly. It can feel to her as if the baby is attacking her. Perhaps it is not only the baby who is gathering dream stuff in feeding, but also the mother. The fantasies that a woman has when her baby is at the breast are an important part of her attitude to breastfeeding. Especially during a night feed, the room in semi-darkness, the world quiet, and when she is only half awake, vivid visual images may impose themselves on her. It is as if dreams have slipped out of sleep and are enveloping her with strange colours, shapes and situations. It is an experience comparable only with fantasies during love-making, involving and growing out of the woman's sense of her own body, its hills and valleys, its boundaries and orifices.

Rich fantasies like this nourish the mother while she is feeding the baby. They form part of her total relationship with the baby and henceforward will always affect the way she feels about her body in all its aspects, even when she has finished breastfeeding and when the baby grows up.

I do not know of any published work on this but women talking about their feelings about breastfeeding often use metaphors and similes which suggest these fantasies: 'I feel like ...', 'It feels as if ...' Problems which the mother faces in her relationship with the breastfeeding baby often disclose themselves in such statements and allow a way to be seen through to a more satisfying experience. When I am giving emotional support to a mother with difficulties I always hope to create a relaxed atmosphere in which she will feel able to talk about these extraordinary body images and fantasies because significant clues are almost invariably revealed.

A woman can do this for herself. She only has to bring these weird shapes and imaginings into the forefront of her mind to be able to see what is making her uncomfortable about breastfeeding, or her whole relationship with the baby, or the sense of herself as a mother. 'I feel parched, drained, dry, a well that has dried out ...' 'It is as if an animal is gnawing at me. I am being eaten up alive ...' 'Like a great mountain, immovable ... completely passive, without life or feeling any more, an enormous dead mountain.' Simple association, allowing the free linking of verbal images and ideas, can take her a long way on the journey towards increased understanding of exactly what she is feeling, and why. But she must put no barriers in the way of the thoughts which come. When such images are blotted out breastfeeding difficulties are often explained exclusively in terms of poor techniques. It is true that the techniques are

often incorrect, but they are so because emotions are inter-
fering with the spontaneous way in which a woman naturally
gives her breast to the baby, and block her capacity to do so.

The mother who just plonks her baby down on her lap,
plugs in the nipple and feeds while staring at the TV screen
or glancing through a magazine is missing a great deal.
There are occasions when a woman feels like doing this and
should feel free to do so. But if she does it habitually she is
not engaging in a relationship with the baby at feed times.
And of course the experience is impoverished for the baby
too. D. W. Winnicott remarked that 'for some babies feeding
experiences are so boring that it must be quite a relief to cry
with anger and frustration which at any rate can feel real,
and must involve the total personality',[9]

The baby who cries 'for no reason' and pulls away from the
breast even when milk is still flowing may be getting the milk
too fast for comfort, but may, on the other hand, be telling
the mother that she should 'switch on' and return to the
scene of interaction between herself and the baby.

There is a stage at about six weeks of age when the baby
first fixes the mother's eyes and holds her gaze while his eyes
grow wider. Some mothers do not 'fall in love' with their
babies until this point is reached. Mothers are well aware of
this important developmental stage when a new social awareness seems to have blossomed, and 'truly social play inter-
actions involving both partners now begin in earnest'.[10]

Transactions between mother and baby progress, becoming more and more intricate, as the baby gives cues not only
about her internal states of comfort and discomfort, hunger
and satiety, but also the objects that catch her attention and
the things she wants to grasp, put in her mouth or bang.

Every game, from peek-a-boo and pat-a-cake to 'Now I
throw it out of the pram and now you pick it up' (irritating as
that one may be for the adult), or 'I pull all the books off the
shelf and you say "No! No!"' and put them all back again,
and I pull the books out again' is for the baby a learning experience and a transaction of this kind.

Babies cannot cope with constant, uninterrupted stimulation, however, and are highly discrimating as to how much they will accept. An adult talking to a baby needs to look away occasionally and give time for him to have *his* share in the dialogue if the conversation is to be continued. A sequence of interaction between a mother and baby is upset, for example, if she goes on smiling continuously and treats the baby as the passive object of *her* performance. She must stop and let the baby have his turn. If she does not, he may turn his gaze away or start to cry, almost as if he could not stand any more. Because she was trying so hard and had evidently failed, she then feels rejected of course. It can become a vicious circle.

Some mothers find it difficult to 'join in the dance' of interaction with their baby because they are very unsure of themselves, or depressed, or anxious, or because the baby is just not the kind of baby they can get on with. An over-anxious mother may consistently over-stimulate her baby, who sends signals to her (looking away or over her shoulder, going glassy-eyed, staring blankly at her as if she did not exist, or even becoming physically limp) which are always ignored. Stern calls this 'mis-steps in the dance',[11] and suggests that when it happens repeatedly we may be witnessing the origins of behaviour that under certain environmental circumstances later develops into 'maladaptive motor inhibitions or passivity as a reaction to interpersonal stress'.

A depressed mother may be unable to give stimulation because she cannot come fully 'alive'. The tempo and pitch of her speech and her movements and facial expressions do not vary much. A baby will then be under-stimulated. Fathers who do not share in baby care and only have a brief session with the baby after coming home from work may have a very limited repertoire of ways in which they can interact with the baby. Although they may play games and put on performances they have not really learned how to have a conversation with the baby. This is a deprivation for the father as well as the baby.

Some babies are ultra-sensitive to stimulation, and if the mother does not modulate her behaviour an amount of stimulation which is fine for another baby will prove too much for him. This may be a factor in the development of childhood autism.

If mother and baby interact in a satisfying way for both, their behaviour becomes *synchronized*. The mother who is feeding her baby and who suddenly notices that he has stopped sucking and is gazing at her begins to talk to him, to wait, as it were for a reply, and to synchronize her speech and action with the baby's activity. The important thing is that she allows herself to be paced by her baby.[12] In fact this synchronization usually comes quite spontaneously to anyone who is relaxed with a baby, who is not anxious to force a response and who is prepared to wait and let the baby initiate conversations of this kind by signalling his attention. Because it begins with the baby's fixed gaze, it is particularly difficult for mothers of blind babies to get synchronized with them in this way. If a baby is in a special care baby unit and having phototherapy for jaundice, as do a large percentage of newborns now, his eyes are bandaged to protect them from the ultraviolet light, and the mother may find it impossible to interact with him.

The baby's participation in sequences of interaction with its mother is an important prerequisite for the acquisition of language.[13] It is partly that the baby discovers that she can elicit behavioural responses from other people by her own efforts to communicate. There would be little point in talking if no one did anything about what one said anyway! It is partly, too, because the very rhythms and cadences of language are linked with rhythms of facial expression and gesture and slight changes in stance or the inclination of the head. The baby is learning this even before the actual words and phrases of spoken language are understood.

When a baby is at the breast interaction between her and her mother takes place spontaneously in between the baby's bursts of sucking. Breastfed babies suck in a rhythm which is different from that of bottle-fed babies. This is not the difference between the bottle and the human breast, but something about the milk itself. Some exciting research in Oxford demonstrates that it is the nature of the fluid being sucked,

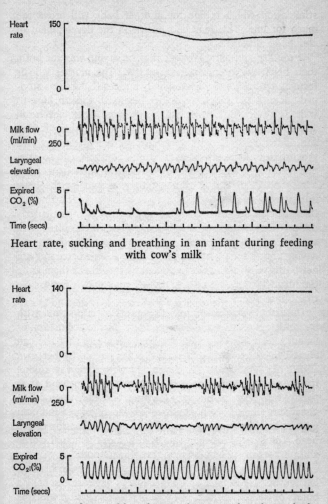

Heart rate, sucking and breathing in an infant during feeding with cow's milk

Heart rate, sucking and breathing in the same infant during feeding with breast milk

Reprinted from *Parent–Infant Interaction* Ciba Foundation Symposium 33 (new series), published by ASP (Elsevier, Excerpta Medica, North-Holland, Amsterdam, 1975.

not the use of the feeding bottle, which produces a different
kind of sucking behaviour.[14] Breastfed babies tend to suck in
bursts, and then pause. They breathe regularly throughout.
Formula-fed babies tend to suck continuously, but at the
same time they often breathe irregularly, and the heart rate
falls at intervals.

In terms of opportunities for creating synchronized behaviour between mother and baby, too, there are in the
bottle-fed baby no spontaneous pauses in which the two
can have a conversation. And because the sucking patterns
are associated with distinctive types of breathing and heart
rate, it is interesting that the synchronization extends, therefore, to *biochemical* levels of interaction between the
mother's milk and the baby.

Feeding whenever the baby seems to want to suck, as
distinct from scheduled feeding, whether at the breast or
from the bottle, provides a valuable opportunity for the
whole process of suckling to become part of a transaction.
The baby asks for what she wants when she wants it, and
the mother responds with milk. The baby indicates when she
likes to pause and when she wants to suck again, and lets the
mother know when she has enough, and she follows the
baby's lead.

A mother who is anxious about the baby or her own
nutritional role, whether she is breast or bottle feeding, may
not allow this transaction to take place. *She* decides that it is
time to feed, treating the baby as a passive container into
which milk must be poured. When the baby pauses, she
jiggles the bottle, or the baby. She may watch the clock and
be determined to get the baby to suck ten minutes at each
side. Sometimes the breastfeeding mother is more inclined
than one who is bottle feeding to try to force the baby to
suck, and to continue sucking without pause, because she
does not know how much milk he is taking and is anxious
that he is not having enough. So we cannot take it for
granted that the woman who breastfeeds interacts spontaneously with her baby in a satisfying way. *The quality of
the relationship is more significant than whether the milk
comes in breast or bottle.*

What we *can* say, however, is that because the breastfed baby is held closely and is in a good position for eye contact with his mother as he is at the breast, because of the necessarily constant interaction with one person, whom the baby gets to know by sight, hearing, smell and touch, and because of the natural burst–pause pattern of sucking human milk, the breastfeeding mother and her baby start off at a definite advantage in this adventure.

16. Sex and the breastfeeding woman

Breastfeeding is one facet of a woman's sexuality. It does not take place in a dimension all on its own and it is to be expected that it affects and is in turn affected by other aspects of her psychosexual life.

In spite of various studies of the subject, no firm conclusions have been reached as to the association between sex and breastfeeding, and whether it increases or diminishes the female libido.

Masters and Johnson found that breastfeeding mothers were more eager to have intercourse again after childbirth than those who were not breastfeeding, and that the uterus returned to normal size and position earlier,[1] and a psychological study of breastfeeding women's subjective estimation of libido in relation to lactation revealed that 30 per cent enjoyed sex more than before the baby was born, while only 2·5 per cent said they enjoyed it less.[2] Another psychological study by David Whitlow in Scotland revealed that breastfeeding 'was associated with a more positive perception of the baby, earlier resumption of sexual intercourse, reduced pain or discomfort and lower sexual nervousness'.[3] Yet many women find that sex is less passionate and becomes more muted and tender while they are lactating, and some are anxious that they are no longer capable of orgasm.

It looks as if the subject is a good deal more complicated than this, and that it is not simply a matter of being 'turned off' or 'turned on' by breastfeeding. There is, after all, not only the woman, but a couple, involved, and the man's feelings about the woman's breastfeeding role must play an important part in this. It is doubtful, too, whether we can look at breastfeeding apart from the context provided by the whole postnatal experience, the ease with which the woman adjusts to motherhood, the nature of her relationship with the baby and her sense of herself as a woman.

I have found that women seeking help for sexual problems
in the first year or so after childbirth always want to discuss
the labour itself, too; they see the kind of birth they had and
the way they were treated then as central to their difficulties.
It may be that it is a convenient crisis on which to focus attention in justification for the difficulties they are facing.
Psychoanalysts would hesitate to accept one fairly recent
event as significant in the aetiology of psychosexual problems. But I know of no studies to indicate that childbirth is
not relevant to how a woman feels about her body afterwards
and in the absence of such evidence it seems reasonable to
accept women's own explanations for what is happening. I
believe we are right to do this anyway because pregnancy
and childbirth are part of a woman's very wide sexuality.

The Kinsey study which claimed to investigate the whole
range of human sexuality never mentioned sex and pregnancy
or sex and breastfeeding. It approached the subject of sex
entirely from a masculine standpoint and concentrated exclusively on genital sex. Yet for a woman sex can be much
more than orgasm and includes a wide range of erotic and
passionate physical experiences associated with childbirth
and breastfeeding.

A grossly lop-sided and male-oriented sex education and
a vast array of publications about sex also neglect these
aspects of female sexual experience. One result is that women
themselves are often anxious that breastfeeding will threaten
their sexuality.

To the anxious woman childbirth itself may be seen as
damaging her identity as a sexual being and bringing with it
the loss of mystery and glamour which both partners may
perceive as important to their sexual relationship. The idea
of breastfeeding may then entail a further de-sexing; she
dreads heavy, hanging, shapeless breasts and envisages nursing as necessitating the release of body fluids in a manner
suited only to the bathroom. It becomes a kind of excretory
function. The man may be anxious too that his wife will cease
to be attractive, that childbirth has altered her vagina and
made it slack, that breastfeeding will intrude on their relationship and, especially if he is unsure of his own libido and

his ability to maintain erections, fear that he will not be a successful lover.

Childbirth itself brings each woman into a dramatic and sometimes distressing encounter with her own body as it undergoes astonishing changes, in a matter of minutes passing through the metamorphosis of delivery to experience an empty body rather than the one that was full of the baby. The melon-shaped bulge of pregnancy is suddenly flat, but also soft, loose, flabby and crumpled. As we have seen in Chapter 3, she may feel vulnerable, aching, bruised, leaking – her orifices exposed, dripping with blood and lochia, and, if she has had an episiotomy, very often mutilated too.

When labour has been a physical and emotional ordeal, or one in which she has been physically restrained by obstetric apparatus, tubes, catheter and wires, the negative feelings about her own body are intensified. Some women report traumatic experiences which may affect their sense of their bodies for ever after:

> ... the final trip to the delivery room ... like a piece of beef ... that side of a cow propped up there on the delivery table ... I remember the doctor and nurse standing between my legs laughing and joking ... thinking, 'I wish I could get out of these straps and belts, I wish I could get off this table and kill them.'
>
> What came back through their conversation was that they were laughing at the mole between my legs on my buttocks. I remember the remark, 'What an odd place for a beauty spot.'
>
> Not only did I hate my husband – the doctor – the whole goddamned institution. But by the time I saw that beautiful baby ... I hated him too.[4]

During the postpartum period the new mother is the object of professional attention and brisk concern. Doctors and nurses ask her about or check her uterus, her bladder, her blood pressure, her bowels and her perineum. They examine the site of the episiotomy and prod her abdomen and her tender breasts. She often feels as if her body no longer belongs to her, but to the hospital. A nurse brings a baby to her and she is handed a bundle containing a strange, squashed, misshapen creature with a receding chin, a brow that slopes back like Neanderthal man, a flat nose and blotchy red marks on its skin, and is told to breastfeed it.

Surprisingly often, mothers are fascinated with their babies, fall in love with them and enjoy cuddling them and putting them to the breast. But it takes no effort of the imagination to realize that given an unloving and alien environment, prolonged separation between mother and baby, a traumatic birth experience or a combination of these factors, some mothers are unable to give themselves to their babies and draw back in the need to protect themselves.

The baby, too, affects the mother's response. One may lie limply showing no interest in the breast, having been drugged by analgesics in labour. The mother who is already uncertain of herself may feel rejected and the baby's behaviour be seen as confirmation that she is not going to be any good at being a mother. Another baby may come to the breast urgently, and the mother withdraws, completely unprepared for the strength of what she sees as an attack, the vitality of this surge of life. Or the baby may seem a raging fury, too angry to feed or be cuddled, and she and it become protagonists in a great struggle to try and get it to take the breast. All these are not simply maternal, but also *sexual* experiences, affecting the way a woman feels about her body and her ability to enjoy and express herself through it. They form part of a pattern of mental images and fantasies about her body and the connection between her body and other bodies, which profoundly influences and is interwoven with fantasies which come into play during love-making. Although some women make an effort to do so because a Puritan morality accentuates the distinction between maternity and sexuality, what happens to a woman's body in birth and breastfeeding cannot be compartmentalized away from her perception of what is occurring in her body during intercourse.

Some women feel very uncomfortable with the sexuality of breastfeeding. It arouses tabooed sensual feelings which they find inappropriate in the relation between mother and baby. Niles Newton[5] has drawn attention to the similarities between breastfeeding and sexual intercourse. Contractions of the uterus occur during suckling and during intercourse. The nipple becomes erect at both times. Breast stroking and nipple stimulation occur in both breastfeeding and love-making. Skin changes associated with vascular dilation and a raised temperature take place in both. The milk let-down reflex is stimulated not only by the baby at the breast but also by sexual excitement. And the emotions experienced may be remarkably similar. Masters and Johnson[6] disclosed that of a group of women who reported feeling sexually stimulated by breastfeeding six out of twenty-four said they felt very guilty about it. Six other women who were not breastfeeding gave as a reason the fact that they had found themselves sexually aroused during breastfeeding of a previous baby.

A woman who cuts off such feelings while continuing to try to breastfeed becomes, in fact, 'frigid' in breastfeeding and, although she may do it from duty, is unable to enjoy it. Almost invariably she has trouble with an inhibited let-down reflex. She cannot allow herself to relax and tends to switch to the bottle after several weeks of unsuccessful breastfeeding.

The nipple, rather than the clitoris, is the part of a woman's body most like the male penis in that it is an erectile, penetrating organ. In response to arousal it becomes erect and must then deeply penetrate the baby's mouth if the suckling is to be a satisfying experience for both mother and child. If it does not enter deep enough, the baby's jaw grips the stem of the nipple and he is unable to draw milk from inside the breast, while at the same time the mother is subjected to pain from the sore nipple. The mother who draws back in this way may be anxious about losing her own strength and vitality; when the milk flows it is as if it were a loss of vital essence. As we shall see, in Chapter 18, she may even say that she feels 'drained'.

This is why an unsatisfactory breastfeeding experience which fails because the woman is concerned to maintain sexual feelings in a separate category of her experience tends to have a negative effect on love-making. It results in the woman being not only exhausted with the effort to breast-feed but having body images which are distorted and ugly. Her body does not work 'for' her as she wants it to. The

sense of inadequacy spreads to encompass the experience of
genital sex too. Whether she acknowledges it or not, the experiences of the body in breastfeeding and in sexual intercourse are inextricably intertwined.

The man, too, may be disturbed by what is in effect a
confusion between distinct categories concerning female
functions in which men have placed women throughout
Judaeo-Christian culture. There is on the one hand the
woman as a sexual being who arouses desire, and on the
other the mother whose love is lavished solely on her child.
Women have been kept in strictly segregated roles of 'harlot'
and 'mother', one despised and the other revered, ever since
Clement of Alexandria said that women were good for only
two things, prostitution and motherhood.[7]

When a woman who excites a man becomes a mother a
man who has been brought up with this view of women, even
if it has not been made explicit, may be unable to respond
sexually to her because to do so would be almost incestuous,
like having intercourse with one's own mother. He is in part
identifying himself with the child, seeing the mother and
baby as if he were himself the baby in its mother's arms, and
demanding that all love and attention is directed to him
alone, uncontaminated by adult sexuality. If the woman attempts to stimulate him sexually he may find it frankly dis-
gusting and be further repelled.

Where this is a cultural theme little can be done to modify
it except through widespread social changes and education
for men and women concerning their relationships with each
other. But when the man is unable to attain or maintain an
erection during the time his wife is lactating it is worth
while for the couple to discuss together his feelings about his
mother and father in their relationship to him as a small
child. He may actually remember occasions when there was
conflict between son and father over the possession of the
mother. Adult sexuality was then, as now, a threat in that it
deprived the child of a mother's love. Yet is this the nature of
love? Is it something which has to be measured out between
members of family, so much here and just so much there? Or
is there not something about the nature of love which means

that it grows and produces light and warmth emotionally enriching to everybody in the family?

LOVE-MAKING WHEN BREASTFEEDING

There is no sexual goal which breastfeeding women need feel they must achieve. Goal-oriented sex after a baby comes is as destructive of real feelings as at any other time. Whether a man and woman are more or less easily aroused while the woman is breastfeeding is part of the rich variation of human nature.

There are, however, special skills of making love during this time, especially during the early months when the woman is living with an unfamiliar body. One cannot just carry on as before.

If a baby has a crying time in the evening, which is very common, a mother becomes anxious. Anxiety is exhausting. When a baby cries intermittently for several hours she needs some time to switch her attention from her baby and 'become herself'. She cannot suddenly be transformed into an exciting sexual creature when she has been walking round with a baby plugged in to her ever since six o'clock. Her husband can run her a bath, make her a drink, tidy up the bedroom, perhaps wash the dishes while she is recovering, then fetch the candles and music.

A woman cannot concentrate on love-making if she knows or even suspects that her baby needs her and may be crying. She can only relax and enjoy her body when she is sure that her baby is contented. Thus love-making is best started just after a feed once the baby has been settled down rather than shortly before one is likely to be given. This is also the time when her breasts are least tender.

Some women cannot surrender themselves to the fantasies involved in love-making when the baby is beside them or in the room. They find they are too tuned in to the baby's needs to be able to focus on their own or their man's feelings. Babies who snuffle and grunt in their sleep, as many do, can be especially disturbing. The baby can be put in another room first or at least tucked behind a screen out of sight.

A woman's nipples may be no longer responsive to sexual stimulation in the way before she was breastfeeding, but respond to the baby only. One who liked her nipples fingered and sucked may no longer find this exciting and the man needs to discover other ways of touching her. If she is still self-conscious about the physical changes produced by pregnancy, such as a soft and crumpled abdomen with stretch marks, the focus of sensation is best created on other parts of the body, such as the small of the back, the upper inside arms, the inside thighs or behind the knees. Any part of a woman's body can become an erogenous zone in the right man's hands. If response to erotic stimulation of the breasts has been lost during lactation, it will return once the period of breastfeeding is over.

If a woman is anxious that she has no sexual feelings while she is lactating it is important to avoid approaching intercourse in any way as if it were a test of love. A woman who finds learning to be a mother a very stressful experience, whose days may be spent in emotional turmoil, may need firm, quiet holding to feel safe before she can allow herself to experience desire.

Love-play may be best started with gentle stroking which is not demandingly sexual. A position in which she is sitting or lying with her back to her husband enables her to get into the rhythms of a sexual encounter without having to demonstrate her erotic response and put on a performance.[8] A man who is anxious about his sexuality while his wife is breastfeeding may also enjoy this approch to love-making.

One of the most important things for a man to remember is that any pressure on breasts full with milk is uncomfortable and that coital postures should be chosen, and new ones experimented with, in which his weight is off his wife's body.

There is more material on sex after a baby comes in *The Experience of Childbirth.*[9]

High levels of prolactin in the breastfeeding woman may prevent ovulation at least in the early phases of lactation. In the Third World prolonged breastfeeding combined with an inadequate maternal diet often contributes to natural child spacing of every two or three years. Taboos on intercourse with a lactating woman further reinforce the use of breast-feeding as a natural means of birth control.

But *breastfeeding is not an effective contraceptive*. Although fertility tends to be reduced during the time when a woman is fully breastfeeding the usual practice in the West of feeding a baby only every four hours makes the early return of ovulation more likely, and it is possible for her to ovulate without being aware that she has, since in five out of every hundred women ovulation takes place *before* they have their first menstrual period following childbirth.

Unless it does not matter to you whether or not you become pregnant again soon, it is therefore unwise to rely on lactation to prevent conception. Up to 15 per cent of pregnancies occur before a woman has had a menstrual period after childbirth.[10]

Some writers suggest that it is safe not to use contraceptives for the first ten weeks if the mother is breastfeeding completely, because only one breastfeeding woman in twenty ovulates before the eighteenth week after delivery.[11] If you decide to do this there is a reasonably good chance that you will not conceive, but it *is* a gamble. Though my fifth baby was fully breastfed whenever she wanted to suckle, with no additional food, juice or water, menstruation returned four weeks after she was born.

Some forethought about birth control is advisable. It is a pity if anxiety about possible conception interferes with the full flood of feeling which many couples experience as they rejoice together in the birth of their child.

The contraceptive pill is inadvisable, certainly before the milk supply is well established, for various reasons. The combined oestrogen/progestogen pill reduces the milk supply,[12] sometimes to dangerously low levels. In some countries, such as Turkey, babies of mothers who are on the pill suffer from starvation. The mini-pill, consisting of progestogen only, does not reduce the quantity of milk, but both kinds of pill may alter the composition of the milk, and research is taking place on this now. Continuing the progestogen pill in the early days of pregnancy may possibly be associated with some kinds of limb defect in the developing foetus.[13] The long-term effects of hormones in the pill on the breastfed baby are not known.

Discuss alternatives with your doctor, at the family planning clinic or in a woman's health group.[14]

You might consider using the diaphragm in conjunction with a spermicidal agent and some women like the original Dutch cap. Neither of these can be fitted until six to eight weeks after delivery. If a condom is used additional lubrication is necessary in the form of a spermicidal agent or other cream (Johnson's K.Y. Jelly, for example) as the moisture normally present in the mucous lining of the vagina during sexual excitement often takes some weeks to return after childbirth. Some women are happy with an IUD, but for many there are unpleasant side-effects, including more or less continual bleeding, and possible long-term consequences are not fully understood.

After a baby arrives many couples discover that sex loses some of its spontaneity. They can no longer make love at any time, anywhere, but have to consider the baby's waking and feeding times. Yet this is made up for by a new closeness and the sensuous satisfaction of being able to lie in bed all three together and marvel that this vibrant little creature was made out of their love. There is a new kind of physical loving to be found in skin contact with a small baby lying against your body, an experience which can be as moving for the man as it is for the woman. Love gains a new dimension.

17. Breastfeeding the older baby

STARTING SOLID FOOD

Any foods other than milk given to a baby will tend to reduce the amount of suckling, and since breast milk is stimulated by suckling the mother may find that her milk supply is
decreased. *Many women can date their gradual loss of breast
milk to the time when they first offered solid food to the
baby.* This is an important reason for not introducing solids
too early, certainly not before four months of age. The baby
needs milk which is designed for and perfectly adapted to its
needs. In the first year of life you cannot give a better food
than human milk, however much care you put into preparing
it. Stuffing minced steak and banana pudding into a five-
month-old may be satisfying for the parents, but does nothing to help the baby.

When it is decided to introduce tastes of other foods there
is a strong case for offering those rich in iron, in combination
with animal protein or natural fruit sugar or honey which
makes it easily assimilable. So egg yolk or prune or apricot
purée are good sources. (Apricots and prunes are usually
sweet enough not to need extra sugar. Never add unnecessary
sweetening to any food or you will train your baby's palate to
expect sweet things.) Baby cereals are often iron enriched,
but can make the baby fat. In a study done at Birmingham
University[1] nearly half the three hundred babies studied at
about the time of their first birthday were overweight and
fifty were classified as obese, being more than 20 per cent
above the weight they should have been. The authors attributed this to giving them cereals far too early in life. When
a baby's solid food consists largely of cereals the child is
sometimes so sleepy and full of stodge that there is much
reduced interaction with the parents and the environment. A

previously bright baby becomes contented and 'good', but in the process stops exploring so actively. It is possible, too, that the early introduction of cereals which contain gluten into babies' diets has led to the sharp increase in infantile coeliac disease over the last twenty-five years, but no one knows for sure.

The argument that you must introduce other foods to 'educate' the baby does not hold water, if only because a great many babies are weaned on to soft, finely puréed foods straight from a can, and cannot get any idea about the variety of real food from this kind of gooey mush. It is not anything that adults and other members of the family eat, but it is a special product called 'baby food'. Yet the only true baby food is milk.

In one advertisement for baby cereal aimed at mothers, two sisters talk to each other; one, who has a bonny, bouncing toddler, exclaiming with shock that her younger sister's baby is not eating 'real food' yet. The younger sister, deeply ashamed, buys a packet of X and gives it to her crying baby who promptly fattens up, gets rosy-cheeked and flourishes. Manufacturers have been quick to see a market in the baby-food industry because mothers want to do the best for their babies and are unsure of whether they are feeding them on the correct diet if they simply mash up food the family normally eats. But provided that your family has a good mixed diet this is the best possible food to introduce once you think that the baby is ready to sample solids.

The sharing of food with others is also an important element in socialization of the growing child.

Foods, through the social and emotional experiences of the context in which they are eaten, become invested with symbolic value and meaning and play a vital part in the socialization of the infant and in his emotional development. However varied the flavours may be, one should ask, what symbolic meaning can an infant derive from a homogeneous food mixture, fed to him in isolation, from a tin which he is not even allowed to examine and play with?[2]

Foods for the older baby can be put in the liquidizer at first, but babies eat such very small quantities that this is

not practicable unless you have a very small liquidizer, such
as one made by the French firm, Mouli, and by some American firms specifically for puréeing baby foods. Or put it
through a manually operated grinder or mill. Keep salt to a
minimum. Babies cannot cope with high salt foods, as we
saw in Chapter 2. Do not be tempted to give your baby stale
left-overs. All food should be fresh. After a few weeks, as the
baby copes with rolling this unaccustomed mess round on
her tongue, you will probably find that most foods can be
adequately mashed with a fork. In most simple societies
mothers chew it in their own mouths before giving it to the
baby.

Some American baby-food manufacturers sent out leaflets
to mothers suggesting that they could poison their babies by
giving them home-cooked food and advised them that they
should buy the company's products instead. Reviewing this,
the Committee on Nutrition of the American Academy of
Pediatrics 'deplores scare tactics' and 'is concerned . . . that
material from scientific publications has been taken out of
context'.[3] It is true that home foods which are puréed contain less vitamin C than commercially produced baby foods,
but this is because vitamin C is added to commercial products. Breastfed babies do not need any extra vitamin C until
solid foods are introduced at about five to six months.
Nitrates are contained in carrots, spinach and beetroot,
which could be harmful if given to babies under four months
old. This is yet another reason for delaying the introduction
of mixed feeding till the baby is about half-way through its
first year. It is not a reason for preferring commercial products to home prepared foods.

The babies of vegetarian mothers who are never given meat
or fish do not suffer any deprivation of important nutrients.
In fact, if the mother is aware of food values they probably
have a better diet than most other babies. Our five daughters
grew up from babyhood as vegetarians and remain so. On the
other hand, it is easy for the first-time mother who is a
vegetarian to lose confidence and feel that she may be doing
irreparable harm to her child. When my first child was about
five months old I took her to a welfare clinic where the

health visitor, checking on this completely breastfed baby's diet, asked: 'You do give her things like minced rabbit, do you?' When I said that I did not and added light-heartedly that I was a vegetarian, she looked horrified and exclaimed, 'Oh, but you must. It is very important or her brain will not develop!' Although I was a reasonably well-informed mother I went home and worried about my malnourished and mentally retarded child. As I write this she has just completed her course in experimental psychology at Oxford.

A lacto-vegetarian will add animal products to her older baby's diet. Vegan mothers, or those who favour a macrobiotic diet, give no animal products at all, however. It is important for them to give their babies vitamin B_{12}. This is added to some vegetable protein products and to plant milks. Proteins can be introduced in the form of ground nuts, cashew nut and almond cream, peas, beans and soya beans. There are also 'baby' kinds of commercial muesli available from health food stores. The Vegan Society produces a booklet on infant feeding.[4]

The Farm, a community in Tennessee, provides good free pamphlets (*Feeding Your Baby Vegetarian* and *Feeding Your Young Vegetarian Child*). Send self-addressed envelopes with redeemable international postage coupons to: Farm Foods, 156 Drakes Lane, Summertown, Tennessee 38483, USA.

WEANING

If you are not under pressure to get the baby off the breast and on to the bottle or cup because work you have to do prohibits continuing breastfeeding longer than a certain time, baby-led weaning is by far the easiest and pleasantest thing to do. But this may mean that you need to have faith that your child *will* ultimately wean herself and will not still be breastfeeding when she is four or five years old!

Signs that a baby is ready for a cup are a great deal of playing going on during breastfeeds, such as undoing your buttons, pulling a zip, springing up and down with her legs, intensive sociability during feeds, or showing evident interest in what you are eating and drinking and trying to share in it. Some babies want to go on sucking much longer than others, and one baby is ready to get all her milk in a cup before the end of the first year of life, whereas another may want to continue at least occasional 'comfort' breastfeeding, at bedtime for example, or before settling down for a daytime nap, into the third year of life. Only you can tell what is right for your baby.

Be relaxed about weaning. You do not have to show you are master and need not be anxious about 'weakening' or 'giving way' to your baby. Follow her lead and make sure that eating and drinking are fun. Above all, do not let implied or outspoken criticism from other people push you into forcing your baby into a pattern which does not seem right for you both.

A mother often says that her toddler is only taking breast-feeds before being tucked up to sleep and that it seems essential for her to suckle to accept sleep happily. Your child is in no way unusual if this is the case with you. Sometimes it is a matter of a good-night cuddle and suckle only, or the breast is a comforter sought when the child is miserable or has had an accident. Some women are rather apologetic about the use of the breast for anything other than 'real food'; but perhaps it is more sensible to be glad that a mother has something to offer her child when he faces the difficult transition between waking or sleep, or when the bottom seems to have dropped out of his world. It is certainly very much saner than putting a child to bed with sticky sweets or a sugary drink, which are bad for developing teeth, digestion and future health.

There are other occasions, too, when some mothers find that suckling suits them as well as the older child. One couple, who were working hard on books late into the night, liked to lie on in bed in the mornings and the only way that their eighteen-month-old would tolerate this would be to cuddle in with them and have a breastfeed. When the mother mentioned this to her doctor he expressed shock and told her that it was bad for her, since she was pregnant, and bad for her little son. But he had no suggestions to offer as to how the parents could have any peace in the mornings otherwise, and when I asked the husband and wife how they felt about it they both, without any hesitation, said how much they enjoyed these times together. It sounded to me as if they had a splendid solution to the problem of an early rising and rumbustious toddler, and one that many other parents, and possibly also the doctor in question, might envy.

There are other women, however, who feel that they need to have their bodies belong to them again. They feel, rightly or wrongly, that tiredness is partly a result of continuing to breastfeed a toddler. (This is not very likely, given a well-balanced diet and good general health.) They may also be very vulnerable to criticism from medical advisers, relatives and friends, who are readily shocked by what may appear to be merely a peculiar aberration of behaviour which smacks of sexual indulgence and 'kinkiness'. There is no reason why you should feel guilty if you decide that it is time to direct your toddler's attentions to milk in cup or bottle or both, rather than you.

It will help a good deal if there is someone else around of whom the child is fond who can give these milk feeds, a person whom the child realizes is not going to offer the breast: a woman friend or relation, or your husband. Cut out the breastfeeds gradually, as with any weaning plan, deciding which you think is the most important emotionally from the child's point of view, and leaving that till last. You are then far less likely to suffer pain from engorgement, which will almost certainly occur if you had a good supply and suddenly weaned, and you may find that your milk will gradually dwindle away.

Make eating times sociable occasions; avoid directing attention to what the child is or is not eating or drinking. A child who refuses to eat when alone may enjoy sharing a meal with a toddler of about the same age. Some mothers find that a new activity introduced at a time when suckling might have been expected is a good idea – 'Listen With Mother' or a swing in the garden or a sandpit. The important thing is to break out of the pattern and for both mother and baby to shake up their routines a bit and start enjoying new things together as the child grows up.

Do not be frightened to refer to the subject of not giving the breast; it will not help to pretend you do not understand the child's request for the breast, if that is what he wants, and can only confuse him. Instead, say cheerfully, 'Not now. We're going to play with the puppets/go swimming/see the cat.'

The decision whether to continue suckling your older child or to offer alternatives is entirely up to you. It does not prove anything about you as a woman or a mother if you choose to continue, or turn you into a more 'normal' or 'successful' human being if you do not. There are no standards to which you have to measure up.

The answer is, of course, that the parents and their baby have to find together a *modus vivendi* and this may be very different from their next-door neighbour's or from anybody else's they know.

Some people who believe that all babies should be off the breast by the time they are a year old still provide bottles, and it is doubtful if there is anything morally, hygienically or socially superior in a child sucking from a feeding bottle than from its mother's breast.

It is sometimes suggested that the mother who engages in prolonged breastfeeding in a culture where most babies are not breastfed for more than a few weeks may be finding it difficult to cut the emotional umbilical cord binding her to her child. The mother may become dependant on her child for her own satisfaction and it is this, rather than the child's need, which is at the basis of breastfeeding into the second or third year of life. In my experience, however, few women are locked in this emotionally dependant relationship and the vast majority of women who breastfeed toddlers and older children are to all intents and purposes 'normal', psychologically healthy women who breastfeed because they think their child still requires it for one reason or another and who want to give their child the best start in life. I used to think myself that lengthy breastfeeding at least hinted at a woman whose fundamental emotional needs were not satisfied, but I have seen no evidence among the majority of those women whom I have met to justify such a conclusion.

Occasionally a woman is bound to a child for personal reasons which counselling may help her to understand. I once met a charming woman who was breastfeeding a three-year-old and a boy of around five, and who did so at a dinner party, but who later asked me if she could have a talk about the stresses which she was undergoing at that time. She told me that she had a prolapsed uterus and her gynaecologist had said to her, 'Right! As soon as you have finished breastfeeding those children we will get your uterus out!' She was continuing to breastfeed in a desperate attempt to put off the evil day and to prolong what she saw as her womanliness. Her problem was that her pelvic floor musculature was extremely slack after two pregnancies and quite difficult births in which no one had taught her how she could achieve active control over these important muscles which support all the pelvic contents. I did not hold out much hope at that late date, but I took the opportunity to teach her some simple exercises for these muscles and we discussed the emotional 'logic' of her continued breastfeeding and the way she felt about her body. A couple of years later I met her again, vibrant with health and joy; she had so toned her muscles that a hysterectomy proved unnecessary and when she realized that she would not have to lose her uterus she was able to stop breastfeeding.

Another woman was suckling a four-year-old; her husband had died tragically just before that baby was born; in her mind she was maintaining a link with the lover and husband she had lost; I suspect that she could not allow herself to face a future in which no one needed her physically. Another woman turned her back on a very unsatisfactory husband, and moved into another part of their large, rambling house for 'peace and quiet' during the time she was breastfeeding, which stretched out, year after year, and effectively protected her from confrontation with a man she no longer loved. These are extreme examples, but perhaps they can remind us that occasionally a woman may be bound to her child and need that child's dependance more than the child may need continued suckling. There is nothing shameful about this; but in reflecting back on the breastfeeding relationship with her child a woman may begin to learn quite a lot about her-self.

When you at last decide that the time has come to finish breastfeeding the severing of that particular kind of relation-ship can be painful for you. This is especially so when you do not intend to have any more children. For it seems as if you are saying good-bye to youth. The door is closing on a whole section of your life which may have been enormously enrich-ing and rewarding. There can be then an emotional crisis which lasts throughout the transition into a life which has other satisfying achievements. The important thing is to recognize that it *is* a transitional period and that you must move forward and you can do something else as well as you breastfed, or better. It is a time when training for a new career, taking up an art or craft you have always wished to have the time to do and developing new skills, can not only be valuable in themselves but can also help a woman over the bridge from being the mother of small children who need her almost undivided attention and concern to becoming a person who is able to offer her children even more than love.

Bruno Bettelheim called one of his books *Love is Not Enough*.[5] A mother is also a *person*. As her children grow up she may owe that to them too.

18. Some social and psychological aspects of breastfeeding

A woman's breasts are not only mammary glands. They form an important part of her image of her body and contribute to her sense of womanliness and sexual attractiveness. Her success or failure at breastfeeding may, depending on her goals, be vital to her feelings of personal worth as a woman and a mother. Whatever her intellectual convictions, the ease and pleasure with which she breastfeeds are in large measure dependant on the way she *feels* about herself and her body after childbirth.

The feelings that she has about her body and the relation between her body and that of her baby through breastfeeding are not just *personal*. They are *social*. The human body and the way in which it is used is part of 'the social construction of reality'.[1]

It is sometimes claimed that a woman with a socio-cultural background in which the female breast is an erotic object inevitably finds it difficult to breastfeed. In our society, certainly, women who believe that the baby's needs come first and who breastfeed in public encounter shocked resistance and may even be ejected from the foyer of an hotel or other public place.

Yet conflict between the breast as an object sexually arousing to a man, stimulation of which is also exciting for the woman, on the one hand, and its nutritional function for a baby on the other is not inevitable. There are many societies in which all mothers breastfeed and where the breast also has an erotic function. The Alorese,[2] for example, solicit intercourse by touching a woman's breasts and a common term for coitus is 'to pull her breasts': 'Our hands move about and touch a girl's breast. That makes her spirit fly away and she has to sleep with a man.' It is incorrect to suppose that in

Third World countries where women breastfeed the breast is perceived only as a lactating organ. It has a dual function.

Breasts have symbolic value for a woman in the eyes of men. The ways in which they are used and the degree to which she is free to do what she wishes with them and to cover or reveal them may also be an indicator of the status of women in society. Perhaps it is significant that the Amazons, warrior women, were said to have amputated one breast and used their exposed torsoes to terrify their enemies as they speeded their chariots towards them.

The power of the mother in the home is given symbolic representation in religious art in the portrayal of a mother with a baby at her breast. Her powerlessness *outside* the home is symbolized by virtually complete covering of the female body, as in Mediterranean peasant cultures.[3]

In nearly all societies parts of a woman's body are hidden by clothing or restricted posture.[4] In some it is concealed in its entirety and even the husband must not see his wife naked. A woman's right to reveal parts of her body, even, in the Arab world, her face, in a public place is severely restricted by powerful taboos and codes of shame and honour. The woman in a Greek mountain village can attain status only as a mother or grandmother in the family. Outside the home she has none. The public world is run by men. The honour of the extended family is vested in the virtue of its women.[5] With rapid social change these codes dissolve, and former taboos, the violation of which brings *automatic* punishment from divine beings, are replaced by laws and injunctions as to female propriety. In Nigeria posters denounce short skirts: 'Long leg is evil . . . Kill corruption.'[6]

When a woman's place in the home is certain, breastfeeding whenever and wherever necessary is readily accepted as being part of the maternal function, and is non-threatening to men. Where, however, male and female roles are changing swiftly and status change brings women into direct competition with men, breastfeeding in public represents a threat to many men that woman is coming out of her hidden place.

In Western culture a female prostitute or stripper is allowed to exhibit her body, and station bookstalls are full of magazines every page of which blossoms with naked breasts, buttocks, exposed belly, crutch and pubic hair, at every possible angle. But this woman is in the category of 'playmate'. Because she is a toy she does not challenge male supremacy. The mother is in a diametrically opposed social category and when she bares her breast to suckle her baby observers may respond with disgust.

When women threaten to escape from these convenient social categories which effectively 'defuse' potential female power, to enter the public arena men, and those women who feel safe and comfortable in these compartments, resent them and feel their own status is jeopardized.

In an anti-breastfeeding culture of this kind the mother who suckles her baby outside the home offends propriety. An Irish journalist attended a chapter meeting of her union taking her baby. When he cried she tucked up her jumper and fed him. At a subsequent meeting she was criticized for doing so by male colleagues, many of them fathers of large families. A father of four exclaimed, with a guffaw, 'But all the same, she has the best you-know-whats this side of Bantry Bay!' and this was followed by laughter and further ribald comment. The discomfort experienced by these men could only be resolved by shifting their image of the woman out of the category of 'mother' and placing her firmly in that of 'tart'.

It is a sad comment on the status of woman and the dignity of nurturing a new life in Western society that such incidents can occur. In Ireland 25 per cent of the population is under ten years, and it seems that mothers must be rather important. Yet in 1978 only approximately 20 per cent of women breastfed their babies.

The mother who casually breastfeeds her baby when and where it wants to suckle is making a symbolic statement on behalf of all women. She may choose to do so discreetly, retaining her right to be 'modest', but she is taking a stand for women as well as for babies.

Yet in the face of these social attitudes, a woman who lacks confidence in herself tends not only to be unable to feed in front of others without self-consciousness, but also to feel,

'How can anything good come out of me?', and this may produce insuperable difficulties in breastfeeding. Distrust in her ability to breastfeed and doubt as to the quantity and quality of her milk inhibit milk production and let-down. In the absence of emotional support these doubts affect also the way in which she handles her baby and offers the breast.

A woman who feels that she has no right to have a baby, to become a mother and, as it were, displace her own mother,[7] may be inwardly convinced that nothing of value can come out of her. The baby's failure to thrive on breast milk becomes proof that it is inadequate, tainted, 'curdled' or 'sour'. It is the woman's image of herself which lies behind such difficulties.

The woman who is pregnant for the first time is passing through a transitional phase in terms of adult female status. She is in a state of 'becoming' in which she grows up out of her status as a daughter to her parents into a new self-image and social status as a mother to her child. She needs to see this assented to in all those round her, but especially her own mother, her husband and the professionals who attend her. It is as if she needs to be given permission to take on this new role by discovering that the 'significant others' in her life find it acceptable and see her worthy of becoming a mother.

If she is treated as just 'a patient' or as a little girl who is acted upon rather than acting, someone who is the passive object of maternity care, there is a very real danger that she may find it difficult to grow quickly enough into being able to cope with the stress of taking on responsibility for her baby. Of course many women survive such treatment almost unscathed and struggle through to breastfeed successfully. But others, more unsure of themselves, are highly vulnerable. They prove unable to interact with the baby in a rewarding way and the result is distress for both mother and child.

Pregnancy and birth, however easy, also entail an abrupt and radical shift in a woman's mental image of her body. At one moment it is full and ripe with child, and at the next it is empty and open. At one moment she is two people, one tucked inside the other; at the next she is a mother having to relate to a strange little creature who is handed to her squashed and crying. Before birth her body is closed, its boundaries containing her baby. After birth it is sagging and leaking, the whole surface damp and sweating, the perineum sore, orifices stretched, tissues bruised and tender, with sticky liquids, it seems, dripping from every opening.

Judaeo-Christian and many other cultures conceptualize the body as a container, the exits and entrances of which must be kept closed except on certain occasions when they are permitted to be opened. To do so at any other time is 'dirty'. As Mary Douglas has shown,[8] matter issuing out of the body orifices is usually considered polluting.

Some women cannot help feeling that breast milk is like an unclean secretion, which, especially because it may stream out unbidden at times which are socially inconvenient in the early days of lactation, is a waste product that has to be cleared away. How can human milk be good for a baby, pure and rich enough to make it grow, when it is a body fluid like sweat, discharged involuntarily like pus or nasal mucus? And the taboo on leaking body substances is combined with a sense of sexual shame at exposure of a part of the body which is normally kept hidden.

Women who breastfeed successfully have been shown to be significantly more tolerant about their children's sex play and masturbation than those who choose not to breastfeed.[9] Attitudes to breastfeeding are part of more generalized attitudes to cleanliness and pollution in the human body.

They also reflect values concerning the relative autonomy of the female body. During pregnancy the mother's body has been inhabited and possessed by the developing foetus. Lady Longford has been quoted in the press as saying (on the subject of abortion) that 'a woman's body is not her own as long as it shelters another life'. It is not just that the pregnant woman may feel that she 'belongs to' her baby but also that in pregnancy mother and baby have been taken over by doctors and nurses. Modern high-technology obstetrics effectively removes from the pregnant and labouring woman any remaining autonomy over her own body. Paradoxically this is occurring at a time when women are increasingly seeking self-awareness and social recognition.

Perhaps this is why some women find trying to breastfeed a distressing experience. To give the breast to the baby is to further extend the period during which the body no longer belongs to oneself. This may be expressed in terms of not wishing to be 'tied to the baby' or of wanting 'to get back to normal'.

In some hospitals today women are subjected to considerable pressure to breastfeed and are denied the right to make decisions about their own bodies. I stressed in Chapter 1 that a woman's freedom of choice is the only basis on which anyone is entitled to give counselling about breastfeeding to mothers. The helper's task is to give full and honest information and emotional support, not to persuade or cajole.

A common reason for not breastfeeding is that the mother has 'never really thought about it' because she lives in a sub-culture within which artificial feeding is the norm. The woman who has emotional support and approval from other family members is more likely to succeed at breastfeeding than one who tries to breastfeed in spite of lack of interest or disapproval from those immediately around her. Women whose mothers have themselves breastfed successfully are influenced by this knowledge to become good breastfeeders themselves. In one study 60 per cent of women who said their mothers breastfed easily breastfed without complementary feeds for eight weeks, wheras only 43 per cent of those who said their mothers did not breastfeed easily were able to do so.[10]

The woman who is socially isolated may start breastfeeding but tends to give up in the absence of support from others in the community. In the USA she is more likely to continue if she has her doctor's encouragement.[11] In Britain, however, she may depend more on the attitude of the midwife who gives her postpartum care and that of the health visitor who maintains personal contact with members of the family throughout the time there is a baby or toddler in the home.

'Caring is the key; that all parents do not feel cared for may be a contributing cause of later pathology in infant and child care.'[12]

But even when there is support from health workers,

women may prefer to bottle feed because the symbolic value of being able to use bottles and artificial formula is great for them. Asian women in Bradford bottle feed although many have previously breastfed babies successfully for two years or more before arriving in Britain. When I asked them why I invariably received the answer, 'Because we wish to do as your women do.' The environment in which they live, which provides a severely restricted view of modern urban society, is that of the northern working class they encounter in their limited excursions outside the home on clinic visits. The acquisition of a brassière and changing to bottle-feeding represents for these mothers an advance away from their peasant past and a way of making their own bodies similar to those of women in the dominant society without surrendering modesty or religious faith. They observe that in this society an object of value is a processed and packaged product involving a money exchange. Those who are most secluded, and who are in *purdah* with the television set, unable to speak English but able to pick up the messages of TV commercials, understand quickly. The only thing that might influence them to consider breastfeeding would be to see English mothers breastfeeding happily, but that is very unlikely in a northern city. No amount of telling them that 'breast it best' is likely to lead to successful breastfeeding unless social influences are brought to bear through cultural contact of this kind.

Commercial pressures in Western society persuade many women that doing the best they can for their babies means spending money on them, and since artificial milk involves expenditure they believe bottle feeding must be superior to breastfeeding. This view is given tacit support by every baby-food advertisement and leaflet for mothers. Preparing for a baby is concomitant with collecting possessions. buying products and equipping the nursery. The bottle sterilizer and other equipment for artificial feeding is seen as an essential part of preparation. Perhaps these women are also saying something about their bodies. They are relatively valueless compared with objects which are acquired. The self is worthy only when decorated and surrounded with artefacts.[13]

. Even when a woman does decide to try breastfeeding, failure of nerve often leads to the introduction of bottles 'just in case the baby has not had enough'. A baby's sucking reflex is usually so strong that she will always take at least a little offered from a bottle following a breastfeed. This is then accepted as evidence that the breast-milk supply is inadequate.

Breastfeeding for a woman today entails a considerable venture in faith, in marked contrast to the manner in which mothers approach breastfeeding in peasant cultures all over the world. Women breastfeed in extraordinarily varied ways. It is perfectly possible to feed a baby with it hanging on the mother's hip, under her arm or slung in a cloth while she pounds grain or coffee beans, or even, as in the Kalahari Desert, to fling an elongated breast over her shoulder to a baby perched on her back! In our own society we make a good deal of fuss about how to position a baby, how long it should suck and how to bring up 'wind'. In spite of this mothers in other cultures are usually more successful at breastfeeding than we are. The essence of this success is that they have self-confidence and are doing something they know how to do in the manner that all other women are also doing in their culture. There is no room for doubt or loss of faith. Breastfeeding is like breathing. You just do it, because nature has equipped human beings to do it.

Mothers in our own Western cultures rarely have such complete confidence in their ability to flow with milk. 'Can milk really come out of my breasts?' 'Is it good enough?' 'Is there enough of it?' 'Surely it can't be real food?' Women may approach the mystery of breastfeeding with the same awe that someone in a technologically simpler society may first witness electricity. And just as in primitive cultures any forces which are not readily subjected to human control tend to be framed round with ritual and magic to ensure that their power is effectively harnessed, so in our own unbelieving culture breastfeeding has produced a whole system of ritual and magic designed to ensure that there is sufficient milk and the baby flourishes.

It also often entails nipple rituals and extraordinarily complicated ways of 'preparing' the breast for lactation, conducting feeds and managing the baby which make of it a highly skilled activity for which the nine months provided by pregnancy may seem to offer inadequate time for training! Breastfeeding has become in our society a task to which the woman has to apply all her ingenuity and intellectual acumen. But while doing all this too often she has never learned how to *let the milk flow*.

We have only to look back at what mothers were taught ten or fifteen years ago to see how ridiculous the instructions often were. Because women had little self-confidence they trusted people to teach them (often middle-aged or quite elderly men) who had not breastfed babies themselves and who had second-hand experience of what it entailed. The experts had frequently never sat with a mother feeding her baby or watched exactly what was going on. Their understanding of lactation was based on medical textbooks and *a priori* principles rather than on direct observation and research. These principles were bound up with a Puritan code of ethics which stated that babies could be 'spoiled' if they got what they wanted and that behaviour permitted in the first days and weeks of life hardened into fixed 'habits' which persisted into later childhood and often into adulthood.

The mother had to start as she meant to go on and above all must show the baby 'who was master'. If she 'gave in' to the baby's crying and fed it at inappropriate times she was 'making a rod for her back'. Consistency was considered one of the main characteristics of the good mother, and if she did not have a plan and a timetable to which she adhered she was in danger of ruining not only her child's physical constitution but also its mental stability.

Mothers no less than their babies suffered inordinately under these systems of management. They often had to listen to their babies crying desperately for food; they lay awake at night listening to the baby screaming in the next room; they were told that the baby must not be picked up except to feed and change it, never just for cuddling, and were warned that doing so would 'over-stimulate' the child who might then become a nervous wreck.

My mother approached the subject of infant feeding from a background in nursing and midwifery and decided that it was more hygienic to bottle feed and that she would follow what was then the latest system in baby care, the Truby-King method. So she had an all-white nursery decorated, the idea being that any speck of dust could be readily seen and that the baby would not be adversely stimulated by shapes, colours or other distractions which could interfere with sleep. I was put into these surroundings resembling a scientific laboratory and my parents were confused and troubled when I yelled and yelled! The books said that I should only be picked up every four hours by the clock, and my poor mother waited in anguish, the nursery door firmly closed, until the clock told her that she could at last pick up her screaming baby. Apparently I cried so much that at last, in desperation, my exhausted parents decided to move me back into their bedroom, where life eventually became easier and where I suspect that mother 'cheated' and, because of close proximity and my ear-splitting utterance, was more inclined to follow her own feelings than the experts' advice.

A great many women went through that experience in those days, believing that they were forging strong characters, assisting the baby's digestion and that letting a baby cry with rage or terror was 'good for the lungs'. The basis was 'regularity'; regularity of feeding and regularity of bowel motions. Tiny babies were sat on a pot after every feed to condition them to empty their bowels into it. Sometimes hot water was put in it so that the steam should act as a stimulant. Nurses prided themselves on having no dirty nappies after the first month. Others triggered off a bowel motion by stimulating the anus at regular times as part of the plan to instil regular habits. It was an extraordinary battle between nurses and mothers trying to follow expert instructions on the one hand and the obvious signals from babies on the other. It is not surprising that husbands escaped from the home and waited until the child was old enough to play trains before getting involved with him.

The new approach to breastfeeding stems from a better understanding of the mechanics of lactation, the baby's nutritional needs and the psychology of the mother as an individual and of her interaction with the baby. It entails drastic modification of the old rules regarding infant feeding, acknowledgement that breastfeeding produces very different patterns of suckling from those involved in artificial feeding, and that the body image of the breastfeeding mother differs markedly from that of the woman who is bottle feeding.

The psychology of lactation is not a matter only of a woman's personal satisfaction but affects the amount of milk produced and may be the decisive factor in success or failure in breastfeeding. When she expresses a positive attitude to breastfeeding at the time of birth she is much more likely to have a good milk supply and to breastfeed successfully. Nearly all the most exciting psychological research on maternal emotions and breastfeeding has been done by one remarkable American woman, Niles Newton. One study of hers revealed that those who looked forward to breastfeeding were nearly three times more likely to succeed in breastfeeding and on the fourth day after delivery provided nearly twice as much milk for their babies than those who did not feel happy about it.[14]

Attitude	Mean amount of milk obtained by baby during feeds on the fourth day (g)	Percentage of successful lactations*
Positive	59	74
Ambivalent	42	35
Negative	35	26

*As judged by no need for bottle supplement after fourth hospital day.

Anxiety, fear and unpleasant distractions can all inhibit the let-down of milk. Niles Newton[15] subjected herself to experiments while breastfeeding her baby and discovered that when her feet were placed in iced water or her toes pulled painfully, and when she had to answer complicated mathematical problems and mistakes were punished with electric shocks, the milk let-down reflex was inhibited. The baby obtained a mean of 1968 g of milk when there were no distractions and only 99 g when there were distractions.

Breastfeeding mothers enjoy body contact with their babies more than those who do not breastfeed. In one study 71 per cent of breastfeeding women said they often slept or rested on the bed with their babies, whereas only 26 per cent of bottle feeding mothers did so.[17] It is imposible to know for certain which is cause and which effect. In mice non-lactating females rescued their pups which had been placed under a sieve eight times more often than mother mice who had had their nipples removed so that they could not lactate. When the mothers had to cross a grid which gave them electric shocks each did so 8·6 times as compared with only 3·5 times with the non-lactating mice.[18]

Studies such as this suggest that successful lactation is part of a specific style of mothering rather than merely a technique at which a woman succeeds or fails.

In the first weeks of breastfeeding many women experience discomfort and pain associated with sore nipples, engorgement, uterine contractions, and even the let-down reflex itself. Research indicates that women who are successful in breastfeeding are just as likely to have pain of this kind as are those who give up. But women who succeed are those who persist, and who for one reason or another are motivated to overcome the difficulties. One of the most common reasons for mothers deciding to stop breastfeeding is that they feel 'used', 'drained', and 'exhausted'. Perhaps what they are really saying is that they feel attacked by the baby, even wounded by it, and that it is drawing life out of them. They resent the fatigue and the feeling that they are being left an empty husk. One has only to watch a healthy, energetic baby snap on to a nipple to realize how readily a mother can feel herself an object of attack.

As we have already seen, a woman who has these negative feelings about breastfeeding is likely to encounter additional physical difficulties. Her nipples may not become erect because breastfeeding does not excite her, just as the clitoris does not become erect if a woman is not sexually stimulated.

The pleasurable rush of heat to the breast in response to the baby's cry, which can be recorded in infrared thermograms,[16] is associated with a sudden, heavy dripping of milk a few days after delivery, but may be inhibited in a woman who finds the idea of breastfeeding distasteful. Not only is the let-down reflex delayed, but breastfeeding is less rewarding and pleasurable for the mother. A vicious circle is created.

It may also be that modern education unfits us for mothering. It is geared towards task-oriented work and to projects which can be completed. Mothering, however, is not like this. It goes on non-stop. Since many a breastfed newborn baby is a more or less continuous feeder, baby care can stretch out in what seems an endless ribbon of days and nights while the mother may struggle to perform 'correctly and by the book', and to get finished tasks which by their nature can never be completed. A mother who is concerned about dust under the bed may never have time to relax and enjoy her baby. One who likes to know that the baby has 'drunk it all up' cannot be satisfied with a method of feeding in which she does not know how much the baby has had or when she will want to be fed again. Where feeding is seen as work there can be no pleasure in the physical contact of breastfeeding.

Mechanical failures and difficulties with breastfeeding at a physiological level cannot be isolated from the psychological aspects of lactation, and psychology is interlocked with social factors concerning the place of women in society. We can only understand why some women face insuperable difficulties in breastfeeding when we know much more about socio-psychological aspects of lactation and see what a woman does with her breasts in terms of men's images of women and women's images of themselves.

19. Ecology, with love

When I was working up in the hills in Jamaica I visited a peasant family, two children of which were in a research project designed to see if giving supplementary milk made a significant contribution to child health. Both these children were in the control group who were to be observed, with their weights, height and measurements recorded only, along with information about their diets. We had to climb up the steep hillside on hands and knees at some points to reach a ledge where the banana-palm-roofed hut had stood, but which had been burned down a few days before. The mother was away 'higgling' in the market, selling crops from the hillside patch she cultivated. Two scrawny little boys were looking after the baby, who must have been about twelve months old, with great tenderness, their only playthings an empty can of sweetened condensed milk, which was the baby's main food, and some sticks and pebbles. The research project doctor examined the baby, who was thin, weak and lethargic and was not growing. As we left he said that he might have to arrange for the baby to be admitted to the university hospital at our next week's visit as it was not thriving and although it was a pity to lose babies from the control group, it looked as if this one would have to have treatment — and food. 'It is always a bit tricky', he added, 'to know exactly when to intervene.'

The following week we went back. The baby was lying in its coffin.

This mother had fed her baby artificially because she wanted to do the best for him and had seen a notice up in the clinic which said, 'Breastfeed till nine months.' With her older children she had breastfed well into the second year of life, but now she understood that the modern thing to do was to put the baby on the bottle so that it was weaned by nine months because breast milk was not good enough from then on. Since she had no access to the special milk supplements which the experimental group in the project had, she gave the baby sweetened condensed milk, which Jamaican peasant children and adults enjoy very much, and because she was poor diluted it in a big jug to eke it out for the whole family. When the level in the pitcher began to get too low she added more water. The bottle she used was a pop bottle which had contained one of the many carbonated drinks which are popular throughout the Western world and this stood around in the heat (I have often seen them covered with flies). Since the dwelling had only one room there was no space for a table and as in most peasant households, there was no family meal. So the baby was not given a share of foods the older members of the family were having, although sometimes the white liquid was thickened a little with cornstarch. The baby cried a lot at first and the mother worried about him, and on the advice of other women gave him herb tea, mint or thyme, sweetened with sugar. This quietened him for a time, but then he would begin crying again. After some weeks, however, he cried less and just lay on some rags in the bath-tub she had put out under the trees and was 'good'. He became progressively weaker and quieter and starved to death.

I think I shall never forget that child. But more important even than this particular baby is the fact that this is happening all over the world and that thousands of other children are dying in this way, or are being permanently weakened and brain damaged by malnutrition during the vital first two years of life.

Simply to say, as do some people who are trying to convince mothers to breastfeed, that one advantage is that the milk 'comes in such cute containers' and another that 'the cat can't get at it' is a very coy approach to the subject and misses the point that breastfeeding has a real ecological advantage. The fashion for artificial feeding which we in the West have set and which, along with the other status-conferring products of industrialization, has spread throughout the world, means that *we* are responsible for these babies being deprived of breast milk.

We are also squandering the world's material resources. If

we consider only the cans and packaging involved in the production and marketing of artificial milk it is obvious that
breastfeeding reduces environmental pollution and conserves
precious resources. An American bottle-fed baby uses 150
cans of formula each year and that amounts to approximately
70,000 tons of tin plate for the nation as a whole each year.[1]
Breastfeeding is something we can still do to correct the
balance between our plunder of our natural habitat and the
life-styles that human beings have evolved.

So breastfeeding is not just a matter of a personal decision
as to what is right for mother and baby. It also has a great
deal to do with the sort of world we want to live in, with
adequate nutrition for rapidly increasing populations and
with whether it is to be survival or death for countless babies
in Asia, Africa and South America. Rapid social change in
Third World countries, above all in developing urban areas,
is associated with declining rates of breastfeeding. In Costa
Rica 40 out of every 100 babies are no longer being breastfed by the time they are four months old.[2] In Fiji 30 out of
every 100 babies are artificially fed by the time they are six
weeks old. In a study done in a village in Mexico it was found
that whereas 91 babies out of every 100 were still breastfed
when they were six months old in 1960, only ten years later
as few as 9 out of 100 were still being breastfed at that age.
In Uganda in 1950 14 out of 100 babies were being given
bottle feeds in addition to breastfeeds and in only five years
this changed until 30 out of 100 babies were being given
bottles. These babies were weaned on average at six and a
half months as compared with fully breastfed babies, who
were not weaned on average till 12·7 months. Whereas in
1951 90 out of 100 well-to-do Chinese mothers in Singapore
started to breastfeed, by 1960 only 70 even began to breastfeed and by 1971 this was down to 50; by the time the baby
is three months old fewer than ten of these mothers are still
breastfeeding. Poorer mothers are even less likely to breastfeed. About 8 out of 100 start breastfeeding, but by the time
the baby is one month old this is down to approximately 5
out of every 100.

In those countries where protein deficiency diseases used to be a special danger for children from about the age of eighteen months, when the staple diet consisted of a high-bulk carbohydrate food with little protein, kwashiorkor, a disease characterized by dry, flaking skin, atrophied muscles and a 'ginger fringe', is now occurring much earlier in life. It was discovered recently in Trinidad that kwashiorkor had a peak incidence at five to seven months, as babies were fed on arrowroot, which, although it looks white like milk, has no protein.

Nutritional marasmus, which occurs when there is a gross lack of calories, not only of protein, and which occurs in the child who is wasting away, is typical of shanty towns on the fringe of urban areas in underdeveloped countries and tends to occur in babies in the first years of life who are fed on much diluted, contaminated artificial feeds. One study of fourteen African countries revealed that over 50 per cent of admissions to hospital for children were because they were malnourished. About a quarter of these children died. These figures did not include the children suffering from respiratory diseases and diarrhoea in which malnutrition played a part, but which were not directly attributable to it.[3]

The problem is an enormous one also in India. In a rural slum where babies were bottle-fed more than 70 per cent of babies under five months old suffered from protein–calorie malnutrition. Up to 60 per cent of babies suffering from marasmus die, and if they do not die there is a high chance of them being permanently brain-damaged.[4]

The cost of artificial feeding is heavy not only for those parents whose babies die, but in economic terms for the country as a whole, a cost which developing nations can ill afford. Alan Berg, consultant to the World Bank, has estimated that bottle feeding in these countries where mothers formerly breastfed their babies is costing up to 1,000 million dollars per annum, without counting the cost of medical treatment for illnesses such as diarrhoea, kwashiorkor and marasmus, which would have been avoided by breastfeeding.[5] In a country like Chile it has been calculated that a herd of

32,000 cattle would be needed to supply the milk which is no longer being supplied to their babies by mothers, over a period of one year (1970). The loss of breast milk in Kenya is equivalent to two thirds of the national health budget.

China is seeing a great return to breastfeeding. Officials there have worked out that mothers are providing the milk for which 100 million cows would otherwise be needed. A Canadian TV film producer told me how remarkably healthy and lively Chinese children were. He had expected to find docile, placid and possibly undernourished children and instead encountered boisterous children who radiated health and vitality. He could not account for it, but the renewed popularity of and government encouragement of breastfeeding may have something to do with it.

THE ARTIFICAL BABY-MILK SCANDAL

When I was in South Africa one of the first things that struck me as I entered Soweto, the African township on the outskirts of Johannesburg, where people live in rows of small concrete huts in a waste of mud, was a massive poster advertising SMA, the 'humanized' artificial baby milk, with an illustration of a fat, bouncing black baby.

Manufacturers of artificial milk have a huge potential market in the Third World and multi-national firms such as Nestlé have gained notoriety for pushing sales among the general public in societies where babies depend on mother's milk for survival. Nestlé is the world's second largest food company, with subsidiaries in twenty-eight countries and the highest sales of baby foods in the underdeveloped countries.

In these societies families are usually too poor to spend money on these substitute milks, and hygiene and sanitation are so rudimentary that bottle-fed infants are prey to gastrointestinal disease and at risk of death. Edward Kennedy, presiding over a US Senate sub-committee on Health and Scientific Research on the marketing practices of babyformula firms in developing countries asked: 'Can a product which requires clean water, good sanitation, adequate family income and a literate parent to follow printed instructions be properly and safely used in areas where water is contaminated, where sewage runs in the streets ...?'[6] Mothers who have no access to a pure water supply or a refrigerator cannot be expected to be able to make up powdered milk which is uncontaminated by bacteria and human and animal waste. It has been estimated that the cost to a poor family of feeding a baby artificially may be as much as 30 per cent or more of its total income. Those who are in extreme poverty dilute the milk so that it lasts longer and eke out a week's supply to last maybe a month. Bottles and teats are left around in the heat with flies and other insects swarming round them.

The only justification for marketing artificial baby foods in countries such as these might be that it is necessary for orphaned babies. When mothers are sick or malnourished there is a strong case to be made for feeding the *mothers* so that they can feed their babies. At present both orphaned babies and those whose mothers are ill are the least likely to get artificial baby milk and simply die.

A survey in Sierre Leone revealed that out of 717 children in hospital because they were malnourished, 713 had been fed on artificial milk. In Chile statistics of infant deaths in 1973 showed that three times as many bottle-fed babies died before they were three months old compared with those who were breastfed.[7]

The scandal of the baby-milk firms was first exposed when an article was published by War on Want, written by Mike Muller, called 'The Baby Killer'.[8] A Swiss organization translated it and published it under the title 'Nestlé Kills Baby', and the firm sued. The judge ruled in favour of Nestlé on a technicality, but added, 'This is no acquittal.'

The baby-milk firms advertise their products by sponsoring baby shows and crawling competitions and use people in nurses' uniforms to promote sales, in much the same way that actors and actresses who seem to have some association with medicine and nursing are used to push the sales of aspirins and vitamins on TV in the West. The difference, however, is that any professional person has superordinate status in a Third World country and an unsophisticated public not used to the conventions of marketing through the media is more easily beguiled and misled.

In 1976 the eleven firms who have the biggest stake in these markets got together to try to work out a code of marketing ethics, but could not come to an agreement. As a result there are now at least three different codes, which in many ways regularize and endorse present practices with minor amendments. For example, one code states that promoters in nurses' uniforms must have the company's badge on the uniform. Some firms, such as Ross, have adopted standards which involve not selling direct to the public and advertising only to the medical and nursing professions. This will not solve the problem of doctors and nurses recommending artificial milks through their own ignorance. In one study in Nigeria it was discovered that 95 per cent of mothers who were supplementing breastfeeding with bottles of formula said they had been advised to do so by a nurse or midwife. Some companies are employing only trained nurses, who are attracted to the work because it is relatively well paid and they get a car, instead of their former 'mothercraft personnel'. But unless these nurses are trained to understand local needs and are loyal to the society they serve rather than the company by which they are employed, this can do nothing to improve matters.

These firms promote artificial milk in hospitals by such measures as providing posters, calendars, diaries and prescription blanks printed with a list of the company's products, and also distribute free samples. Governments in the Third World are becoming increasingly alarmed about such activities. Papua/New Guinea has banned all advertising of artificial milk except to health workers and the sale of formula and bottles without a health worker's prescription. But unstable governments are often powerless compared with the strength of these multi-national companies, and clinics and hospitals frequently lend implicit support to big business by accepting gifts such as refrigerators and other equipment and in return allowing promotion of company products to take place in the hospital. Hospital staff may not see it as a business deal, but in effect it is. Representatives from these firms are often allowed to promote artificial milk to expectant and newly delivered mothers waiting in the clinics and even have access to their bedsides.

A few of these companies have responded positively to public disquiet by a brave decision to discontinue advertising in underdeveloped countries unless their advertising material has been approved by paediatricians in those countries. As a result Cow and Gate have had to cancel some contracts and allow others to lapse.

But none of these new codes of practice, however bold, can be enforced; they depend on the determination of the firms' own management to abide by such a policy. Moreover, some of the statements of intention are virtually contradictory. It is difficult for a sales woman to avoid 'discouraging mothers from establishing or continuing breastfeeding', as stated in the code of ethics of the International Council for Infant Food Industries, when she is employed to promote the sales of artificial milk. Only when there is a ban on sales agents giving any advice to mothers and when there are statutory controls on the advertising of artificial baby foods similar to those on the advertising of cigarettes shall we be on the way to giving social approval to breastfeeding.

IMMIGRANT MOTHERS

In our own society artificially fed babies are not exposed to the risks of those in the underdeveloped countries. But it is not so long ago that bottle-fed babies in the West were subjected to just the kind of dangers that those in the Third World face today. Before refrigerators were available babies were considered especially vulnerable during the second summer of their lives, when they were off the breast, and especially if they lived in a city getting possibly contaminated milk from cows who were kept in the basements of breweries so that they could be fed on the by-products of beer; the milk was put in pails and hawked in the street. My mother described to me how seventy years ago she remembers the 'bubby pot' (feeding cup) containing pap or bread soaked in cow's milk and the baby's bottle from which a long tube projected, finishing in a teat, both kept permanently at the side of the coal range, warm and ready to quieten a fractious toddler or infant. This was a period when mothers spoke proudly of having borne twelve children and reared nine, as mothers do today in the underdeveloped countries.

A much improved standard of living, better housing, easy access to water, modern sewage, facilities for sterilizing bottles and teats, and refrigerators have changed all this. Asian mothers who choose to bottle feed their babies when they emigrate to Britain, do so very successfully and their babies flourish. It is surprising how quickly child-rearing styles can change, for these same women have often breast-fed babies before for two to three years. But as we have seen, this is a conscious adjustment to the life-style of the dominant society. Caribbean women in Britain are more likely to breastfeed and continue a mixture of breast and bottle feeding while they go back to work. Although combined breast and bottle feeding does not seem to work well for women who fear they have too little milk (the most frequent reason for resorting to this method of feeding) with women who see it as the only way of continuing breastfeeding when they return to employment outside the home it seems to work, and they give frequent breastfeeds before and after returning from work and during the night if the baby wakes.

Economic reasons often drive a woman outside the home at a time when her baby needs her. Some mothers may find a partial solution in giving as much time to their babies as possible when they are at home. But to switch from breast to bottle may be to deprive a baby not only of its mother's milk but also of the closeness and caring that is associated with holding it to the breast, especially when this closeness, because it cannot be measured or statistically evaluated, has never reached the headlines of our newspapers and cannot be taught in mothercraft or home economics lessons. A psycho-analyst friend of mine remembers with horror being in a big London maternity hospital after her daughter was born and the Sister coming to the ward early each evening, clapping her hands for attention, and calling: 'Now ladies! Pick up your babies! Mothering time!'

Perhaps the undervaluing of the mother–child relationship in our society is responsible in large measure for loving immigrant mothers seeking baby-minders and foster homes so that they can study and earn to provide the child with material goods in the future. Those advertisements for 'kind, clean foster mothers' and whole-day minders on newsagents' doors reflect values inherent in our own society. They are the logical extension of a faith in technical achievements and professional knowledge rather than in a mother's capacity to give her baby a special and unique experience which is mutually enriching.

For society to give support to breastfeeding it is not enough to encourage mothers through health education programmes to nurse their babies, nor even enough to have rooms where mothers can breastfeed in comfort in all large stores and in stations, airports and other public places. Much more radical reorganization is required. In 1977 the British Trades Union Congress passed unanimously a resolution proposed by the Health Visitors' Association:

Congress notes with concern the wastage of one of the most important natural resources – human breast milk; and calls upon the Government to consider and implement ways in which all mothers may be given the choice to breastfeed their babies, and urges the following measures:

(a) An on-going campaign to promote breastfeeding which at least matches in size and strength that of the sales promotion and advertising efforts of the commercial baby-milk manufacturing industry:

(b) Greater flexibility in the timing of the payment of the weekly state maternity allowance to enable mothers to draw benefit for a longer period after the birth of their babies and thus maintain breastfeeding;

(c) More facilities so that women may continue to breastfeed during the working day after returning to employment.

Such a resolution may be only a straw in the wind, but it does suggest that we are beginning to recognize the importance of breastfeeding and at least to ask why it should be impossible to make the necessary social changes for it to be done more generally. The Health Visitors' Association is collecting evidence about arrangements and work-place facilities for breastfeeding women in other countries and in the United Kingdom. It is interesting that although they are finding it easy to obtain information about what is offered in East Germany, China and the Soviet Union, countries where women in employment get time off during working hours in which to breastfeed, they are unable to get information about similar arrangements in the United Kingdom.

The importance of breastfeeding will only be recognized adequately when all work-places (shops, factories, schools, hospitals, offices) provide facilities for breastfeeding, have nurseries in which babies can be close to their mothers at work and give women time off to breastfeed. That, in turn, means a rethinking of the importance of the woman in her role as a mother in the modern world and, perhaps equally, a rethinking of the roles of men as fathers too.

Addresses of helpful organizations

The National Childbirth Trust, 9 Queensborough Terrace, Bayswater, London. W2 3TB (tel. 01 229 9319/9310). The Breastfeeding Promotion Group gives mother-to-mother help with breastfeeding. Local Postnatal Support Groups offer peer group emotional support from other mothers.

La Leche Great Britain, Box 3424, London, WC1 6XX. Gives help and advice on breastfeeding. You will be given a local phone number.

Breast pumps can be obtained through the National Childbirth Trust from Barbara Tapling (the Kaneson hand pump), The Elms, Church Meadow Lane, Heswall, Merseyside (tel. 151 342 6638) – this small hand pump is useful once the milk supply is well established if you have to miss a feed; and Sheila Smith (the Engell electric pump), 26 Lyndhurst Gardens, Finchley, London N3 – this pump is useful if your baby is in special care and you want to build up your milk supply.

The Lact-Aid can be obtained from La Leche at the above address, or through the NCT from Judy Morrison, 97 Camden Road, London NW1 (tel. 01 267 2870).

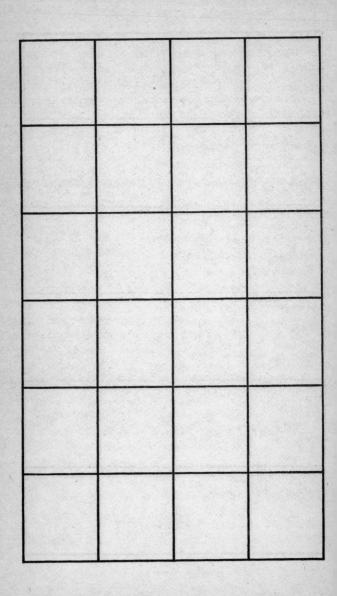

Notes

1. LEARNING ABOUT BREASTFEEDING

1. W. H. Masters and V. E. Johnson, *Human Sexual Response*, Boston, Little, Brown, 1966; and *Human Sexual Inadequacy*, Boston, Little, Brown, 1970.

2. IS HUMAN MILK GOOD ENOUGH FOR BABIES?

1. P. R. Payne and Erica F. Wheeler, 'Comparative nutrition in pregnancy and lactation', *Proceedings of Nutrition Society*, 1967.

2. Derrick B. Jelliffe and E. F. Patrice Jelliffe, *Human Milk in the Modern World*, London, OUP, 1978. This is the modern classic on lactation and much of the scientific data in this chapter is derived from this book.

3. Jelliffe and Jelliffe, op. cit.

4. Paul Buisseret, 'Common manifestations of cow's milk allergy in children', *Lancet*, 8059, 304–5, 1978.

5. B. Hall, 'Changing composition of human milk and early development of an appetite control', *Lancet*, 7910, 779–81, 1975.

6. Christopher Rolles, Mabel Liddiard Memorial Lecture, reproduced in *Nursing Mother's Association of Australia Newsletter*, 12 (6), 1–7, 1976.

7. Rolles, op. cit.

8. Rolles, op. cit.

9. W. H. Whittlestone, 'The value of human milk', *Parents' Centres Bulletin*, 70, Federation of New Zealand Parents' Centres Inc., 1977.

10. R. Reiser and Z. Sidelman, 'Control of serum cholesterol homeostasis by cholesterol in the suckling rat', *Journal of Nutrition*, 102, 1009, 1972.

11. Jelliffe and Jelliffe, op. cit.

12. Jelliffe and Jelliffe, op. cit.

13. Whittlestone, op. cit.

14. D. R. Lakdawala and E. M. Widdowson, 'Vitamin D in human milk', *Lancet*, 1,8004, 167, January 1977.

15. D. P. Davies and R. Saunders, 'Blood urea: normal values in early infancy related to feeding practices', *Archives of Diseases of Childhood*, 48, 563, 1973.

16. M. G. Philpott, 'Infant foods and softened water', *Lancet*, i, 1378, 1975.

17. H. McKay, 'Anaemia in Infancy', *Archives of Diseases in Childhood*, 3, 1175, 1926.

18. J. A. McMillan, S. A. Landaw and F. A. Oski, 'Iron sufficiency in breastfed infants and the availability of iron from human milk'. *Pediatrics*, 58, 686. 1976.

19. V. M. Saarinen and others, 'Iron absorption in infants', *Journal of Pediatrics*, 1, 36–9, 1977.

20. L. M. Klevay, 'The ratio of zinc to copper in milk and mortality due to coronary heart disease', in *Trace Substances in Environmental Health*, Vol. VIII (D. D. Hamphill, ed.), Columbia University of Missouri, 1974.

21. E. F. P. Jelliffe, 'Infant feeding practices, associated iatrogenic and commerciogenic diseases', *Pediatric Clinics of North America*, 24, 1, 49, 1977.

22. L. S. Hurley, 'Zinc deficiency in prenatal and neonatal development', in G. J. Brewer and A. S. Prosod, eds., *Zinc Metabolism: Current Aspects in Health and Disease*, New York, Alan R. Liss Inc., 1977.

23. P. D. Buisseret, op. cit.

24. Buisseret, op. cit.

25. June Clark, 'The baby-milk controversy', *Nursing Mirror*, 26 February 1976.

26. London, HMSO, 1974.

27. Walter Whittlestone, comparative mammologist working at Ruakura Agricultural Research Centre, New Zealand; personal communication.

28. L. A. Hanson and J. Winberg, 'Breastmilk and defence against infection in the newborn', *Archives of Diseases of Childhood*, 47, 845, 1972.

29. P. A. Gyorgy, 'Biochemical aspects of human milk', *American Journal of Clinical Nutrition*, 24, 976, 1971.

30. C. L. Bullen and A. T. Wills, 'Resistance of the breast fed infant to gastroenteritis', *British Medical Journal*, 3, 338, 1971.

31. Walter Whittlestone, personal communication.

32. A. S. Cunningham, 'Morbidity in breast fed and artificially fed infants', *Journal of Pediatrics*, 5, 726–9, 1977.

4. THE BREAST

1. Marvin E. Eiger and Sally Wendkos Olds, *The Complete Book of Breastfeeding*, London, Bantam, 1973.

2. Personal communication.

3. W. H. Masters and V. E. Johnson, *Human Sexual Response*, Boston, Little, Brown, 1966.

4. R. Applebaum, 'Breastfeeding and care of the breasts', *Davis' Gynecology and Obstetrics*, Vol. I, New York, Harper & Row, 1974.

5. THE MOMENTOUS HOUR AFTER BIRTH

1. *The Psychology of Childbirth*, London, Fontana, 1977.
2. Marshall Klaus and John Kennell, *Maternal–Infant Bonding*, St Louis, Mosby, 1976.
3. Dotti Rees, 'Breastfeeding the premature infant', *Keeping Abreast Journal*, II, 2, 1977.
4. Rudolph Schaffer, *Mothering*, London, Fontana, 1977.

7. THE HOSPITAL

1. See *The Good Birth Guide*, London, Fontana, 1978.
2. I. Chalmers, H. Campbell and A. C. Turnbull, 'Use of oxytocin and incidence of neonatal jaundice', *British Medical Journal*, III, 1975; I. Chalmers, 'Neonatal jaundice', *Nursing Times*, July 1976.
3.–Marshall H. Klaus and John H. Kennell, *Maternal–infant Bonding*, St Louis, Mosby, 1976.

8. THE BABY

1. *Birth without Violence*, London, Wildwood House, 1975.
2. A. Janov, *The Primal Scream*, London, Sphere Books, 1973;
3. J. B. Brazleton, 'Effects of maternal medication on the neonate and his behaviour', *Journal of Pediatrics*, 58, 513, 1961.
4. R. E. Kron, M. Stein and K. E. Goddard, 'Newborn sucking behaviour affected by obstetric sedation', *Pediatrics*, 37, 1012–16, 1966.
5. W. A. Bowes, Y. Brackbill and A. Steinschneider, 'The effects of obstetrical medication on fetus and infant', *Monographs Social Research and Child Development*, 35, 4, 1970.
6. Marshall H. Klaus and John H. Kennell, *Maternal–Infant Bonding*, St Louis, Mosby, 1976.
7. A. Blake, A. Stewart and D. Turcan, 'Parents of babies of very low birthweight: long term follow-up', in R. Porter and M. O'Connor, eds., *The Parent–Infant Relationship* (Ciba Foundation Symposuim), Amsterdam, Elsevier, 1974.
8. Klaus and Kennell, op. cit.
9. 9 Queensborough Terrace, London W2 3TB.

9. SLEEPING, WAKING AND CRYING

1. *Birth Without Violence*, London, Wildwood House, 1975.
2. A. H. Parmelee, W. H. Wenner and H. R. Schulz, 'Infant sleep patterns from birth to 16 weeks of age', *Journal of Pediatrics*, 65, 576–82, 1964.
3. J. A. Ambrose, ed., *Stimulation in Early Infancy*, London and New York, Academic Press, 1970.

4. J. and B. Tizard, 'The social development of two-year-old children in residential nurseries', in H. R. Schaffer, ed., *The Origins of Human Social Relations*, London, Academic Press, 1971.

5. John Bowlby, *Attachment*, Penguin Books, 1971.

6. Yvonne Brackbill, 'Cumulative effects of continuous stimulation on arousal level in infants', *Child Development*, 42, 17–26, 1971.

7. Sheila Kitzinger, *Women as Mothers*, London, Fontana, 1978.

8. It is available at a reduced price through the NCT, 9 Queensborough Terrace, London W2 3TB.

9. *Mothering*, London, Fontana, 1977.

10. Sheila Kitzinger, Penguin Books, 4th ed., 1978.

10. DIFFICULTIES

1. Ilene Rice, *Heartstart*, St Paul, Minnesota, privately published, 1978.

2. *Keeping Abreast Journal*, Vol. I, 2, 1976.

3. Marvin S. Eiger and Sally Wendkos Olds, *The Complete Book of Breastfeeding*, London, Bantam, 1973.

4. Dotti Rees, 'Sore nipples are a pain!', *Keeping Abreast Journal*, Vol. I, 2, 1976.

5. W. H. Whittlestone, 'The value of human milk', *Parents' Centres Bulletin*, 70, Federation of New Zealand Parents' Centres Inc., 1977.

6. W. H. Whittlestone, op. cit.

7. Bryne R. Marshall, James K. Hepler and Clyde C. Zirbel 'Sporadic puerperal mastitis: an infection that need not interrupt lactation', *Journal of the American Medical Association*, 233, 1577–9, 1976.

8. M. Ounsted, 'Infant feeding', *Nursing Times*, 6 May, 1976.

9. I am grateful for advice from Dr J. D. Baum of the Radcliffe Infirmary, Oxford, on this subject.

10. D. L. Miller, 'Birth and long-term unsupplemented breastfeeding in seventeen dependant diabetic mothers', *Birth & The family Journal* 4, 2, Summer 1977.

11. J. E. Tyson and R. A. Hock, 'Gestational and pregestational diabetes: an approach to therapy', *American Journal of Obstetrics and Gynecology*, 125, 7, 1009, 26 August 1976.

12. M. J. Brothers, *Diabetes: The New Approach*, Crosset & Dunlap, 1976.

11. CRISIS

1. David W. Hide, 'Hypoglycaemia in the newborn infant', *Maternal & Child Care*, August 1967; P. A. Davies and J. P. Davies, 'Very low birth weight and subsequent head growth', *Lancet*, 2, 1216–19, 1970.

2. Sheila Kitzinger, *The Good Birth Guide*, London, Fontana, 1978.

3. *The Tender Gift: Breastfeeding*, New York, Prentice-hall, 1973.

4. Personal communication

5. J. L. Avery, *Induced Lactation*, J. J. Avery Inc. See page 227 for addresses from which the Lact-Aid can be obtained.

6. See page 227.

7. See *Keeping Abreast Journal,* Vol. I, 2, 1976.

8. A mother whose baby had a diaphragmatic hernia. *Keeping Abreast Journal,* Vol. I, I, 1976. See Janice Nau, 'When a nursing baby has surgery' in the same issue.

9. Niles Newton and Marilyn Theokatos, 'Problems and satisfactions of over 600 women who breastfed during pregnancy', 5th International Congress of Psychosomatic Obstetrics and Gynaecology, Rome, 1977.

12. EVERYBODY ELSE IS COPING; WHY CAN'T I?

1. *Normality and Pathology in Childhood,* Penguin Books, 1973.

2. London, Severn House, 1977.

13. BREASTFEEDING IN A POLLUTED WORLD

1. World Health Organization, *Pesticide Residues in Food,* Report of 1970 Joint FAO/WHO Meeting, Technical Reports series, 474, 1971.

2. Reported in *New York Times,* 20 September 1977.

3. Derrick B. Jelliffe and E. F. Patrice Jelliffe, *Human Milk in the Modern World,* London, OUP, 1978.

4. E. M. Widdowson, J. E. Slater, G. E. Harrison and A. Sutton, 'Absorption and retention of strontium by breast-fed and bottle-fed babies', *Lancet,* 2, 941, 1960.

5. D. G. Mitchell, 'Increased lead absorption: paint is not the only problem', *Pediatrics,* 53, 142, 1974.

6. I. Chalmers, H. Campbell and A. C. Turnbull, 'Use of oxytocin and incidence of neonatal jaundice', *BMJ,* ii, 116, 1975; T. Hargreaves and R. F. Piper, 'Breast milk jaundice', *Archives of Diseases of Childhood,* 46, 195, 1971; A. P. Cole and T. Hargreaves, 'Conjugation inhibitors and early neonatal hyperbilirubinaemia', *Archives of Diseases of Childhood,* 47, 415, 1972.

7. Roy Ing, J. H. C. Ho and N. L. Petrakis, 'Unilateral breastfeeding and breast cancer', *Lancet,* ii, 8029, 1977.

8. J. F. Fraumeni and R. W. Miller, 'Breast cancer from breast feeding', *Lancet,* ii, 1196, 1971.

9. Jelliffe and Jelliffe, op. cit.

10. This and much of the following information is obtained in: Paula C. Rothermel and Myron M. Faber, 'Drugs in breastmilk – a consumer's guide', *Birth and the Family Journal,* Vol. 2, 3,

11. op. cit.

12. Penny and Andrew Stanway, *Breast is Best,* London, Pan Books, 1978.

13. M. Fowler, 'A new era in breastfeeding', *Journal Pediatrics,* 22, 34, 1976.

14. Richard M. Applebaum, 'Breastfeeding and drugs in human milk', *Keeping Abreast Journal*, 2, 4, 1977.

15. *Federal Register*, 41, 115, 14 June, 1976.

16. Mary White, *Breastfeeding and Drugs in Human Milk*, La Leche Information Sheet.

17. Applebaum, op. cit.

14. THE FOOD YOU EAT

1. A. Chavez and others: 'Role of lactation in the nutrition of low socioeconomic groups', *Ecology of Food and Nutrition*, 4, 1959, 1975.

2. Dietary Standard for Canada.

3. Frances Moore Lappé, New York, Ballantine, 1971.

4. Gaynor D. Maclean, 'An appraisal of the concepts of infant feeding and their application in practice', *Journal of Advanced Nursing*, 2, pp. 111–26 (Blackwell Scientific Publishers, Oxford, 1977).

15. COMMUNICATION AND RELATIONSHIPS

1. Aidan Macfarlane, *The Psychology of Childbirth*, London, Fontana, 1977.

2. Genevieve Carpenter, 'Mother's face and the newborn', *New Scientist*, 742–4, 21 March, 1974.

3. C. and S. J. Hutt, 'Auditory discrimination at birth', in S. J. and C. Hutt, eds., *Early Human Development*, London, O U P, 1973.

4. 'Olfaction in the development of social preferences in the human neonate', *Parent–Infant Interaction*, Ciba Symposium 33, Amsterdam, Elsevier, 1975.

5. P. M. Stratton, 'Criteria for assessing the influence of obstetric circumstances on later development', Tim Chard and Martin Richards, eds., *The Benefits and Hazards of the New Obstetrics*, Spastic International Medical Publications, 1977.

6. Daniel Stern, *The First Relationship: Infant and Mother*, London, Fontana, 1977.

7. H. F. R. Prechtl, 'Problems of behavioural studies in the newborn infant', in D. S. Lehoman, R. A. Hindle and E. Shaw, eds., *Advances in the Study of Behaviour*, London and New York, Academic Press, 1965.

8. J. Newson, 'Towards a theory of infant understanding', *Bulletin of the British Psychological Society*, 27, 251–7, 1974.

9. In a talk given to the National Childbirth Trust, 1969.

10. Daniel Stern, op. cit.

11. Daniel Stern, op. cit.

12. H. R. Schaffer, ed., *Studies in Mother–Infant Interaction*, London, Academic Press, 1977.

13. J. S. Bruner, 'The ontogenesis of speech activities', *Journal of Child Language*, 2, 1–19, 1975.

14. P. Johnson and D. M. Salisbury, 'Breathing and sucking during feeding in the newborn', *Parent–Infant Interaction*, Ciba Foundation Symposium 33, Amsterdam, Elsevier, 1975.

16. SEX AND THE BREASTFEEDING WOMAN

1. William H. Masters and Virginia E. Johnson, *Human Sexual Response*, Boston, Little, Brown, 1966.
2. Alice K. Ladas, 'How to help mothers breastfeed: deductions from a survey', *Clinical Pediatrics*, 9, 702–5, 1970.
3. Personal communication.
4. B. Cowan, ed., *Death of the Deity*, quoted in James E. and Jane G. Pittenger, 'The perinatal period: breeding ground for marital and parental maladjustment', *Keeping Abreast Journal*, 2, 1, 1977.
5. 'Interrelationship between sexual responsiveness, birth and breastfeeding', in *Contemporary Sexual Behaviour*, J. Zubin and J. Money, eds., Baltimore, John Hopkins Press, 1973.
6. Masters and Johnson, op. cit.
7. See Sheila Kitzinger, *Women as Mothers*, London, Fontana, 1978.
8. Helen Singer Kaplan, *The New Sex Therapy*, London, Ballière Tindall, 1974, W. H. Masters and Virginia E. Johnson, *Human Sexual Inadequacy*, Boston, Little Brown, 1970.
9. Sheila Kitzinger, Penguin Books, 4th ed., 1978.
10. Derrick B. Jelliffe and E. F. Patrice Jelliffe, *Human Milk in the Modern World*, London, OUP, 1978.
11. Penny and Andrew Stanway, *Breast is Best*, London, Pan Books, 1978.
12. See Chapter 13.
13. Jelliffe and Jelliffe, op. cit.
14. Addreses of these are often given in *Spare Rib* or can be obtained at a Citizens' Advice Bureau or city information centre. See also *Our Bodies Our Selves*, by the Boston Women's Health Collective, Penguin Books, 1978.

17. BREASTFEEDING THE OLDER BABY

1. A. Shukla, H. A. Forsyth, Charlotte M. Anderson, S. M. Marwah, 'Infantile overnutrition in the first year of life', *British Medical Journal*, Vol IV, pp. 507–15, 1972.
2. E. H. Hipsley, 'One of the family – do children need special foods?' *Parents' Centres Bulletin*, 70, 1977, New Zealand.
3. *News & Comment*, American Academy of Pediatrics, 11, 2, 11, 1976.
4. *Vegan Mothers and Children*, The Vegan Society, 47 Highlands Road, Leatherhead, Surrey.
5. New York, Free Press, 1959.

18. SOME SOCIAL AND PSYCHOLOGICAL ASPECTS OF
BREASTFEEDING

1. Peter L. Berger and Thomas Luckmann, *The Social Construction of Reality* Penguin Books, 1971.

2. Seymour Fisher and Sidney E. Cleveland, *Body Image and Personality*, New York, Dover, 1968.

3. Sheila Kitzinger, *Women as Mothers*, London, Fontana, 1978.

4. Ted Polhemus, ed., *Social Aspects of the Human Body*, Penguin Books, 1978.

5. Sheila Kitzinger, op. cit.

6. Polhemus, op. cit.

7. Sheila Kitzinger, *The Experience of Childbirth*, Penguin Books, 4th ed. 1978.

8. *Purity and Danger*, Penguin Books, 1970.

9. R. R. Sears, E. E. Maccoby and H. Levin, *Patterns of Child Rearing*, Evanston, Row, Petersen, 1957.

10. M. Newton, 'Human lactation', in S. K. and A. T. Cowie, eds., *Milk: The Mammary Gland and Its Secretion*, Vol. I, New York, Academic Press, 1961.

11. Kathleen G. Auerbach, 'To breastfeed or not to breastfeed', *Keeping Abreast Journal*, I, 4, 1967.

12. Auerbach, op. cit.

13. See Erving Goffman, *The Presentation of Self in Everyday Life*, Penguin Books, 1971.

14. Niles and Michael Newton, 'Psychologic aspects of lactation', *New England Journal of Medicine*, 277, 1179, 1967.

15. Michael and Niles Newton, 'The let-down reflex in human lactation', *Journal of Pediatrics*, 33, 698–704, 1948.

16. J. Lind, V. Vuorenkoski and O. Wasz-Höckert, 'The effect of cry stimulus on the temperature of the lactating breast of the primipara', in N. Morris, ed., *Psychosomatic Medicine in Obstetrics and Gynaecology*, Basle, Karger, 1972; O. Wasz-Höckert, Leila Setamo, V. Vuorenkoski, T. Partanen and J. Lind, 'Emotional attitudes toward the child and child rearing and the effect of the cry stimulus on the skin temperature of the lactating breast in primiparas', in Morris, op. cit.

17. N. Newton, D. Peeler and C. Rawlins, 'Does breastfeeding influence mother love? An experimental and statistical study on mouse and man', in Morris, op. cit.

18. N. Newton, D. Peeler and C. Rawlins, 'Effect of lactation on maternal behaviour in mice with comparative data on humans', *Journal of Reproductive Medicine*, 1, 257–72, 1968.

19. ECOLOGY, WITH LOVE

1. Derek B. Jelliffe and E. F. Patrice Jeliffe, *Human Milk in the Modern World*, London, OUP, 1978.

2. For this and subsequent material on the world scene see Jelliffe and Jelliffe, op. cit, an excellent source of information on baby-feeding practices throughout the world.

3. K. V. Bailey, 'Malnutrition in the African Region', *World Health Chronicle*, 29, 354, 1975.

4. John Dobbing, 'Nutrition and the developing brain', letter in *Lancet*, i, 48, 1973.

5. Alan Berg, *The Nutrition Factor*, Washington, Brookings Institute, 1973.

6. 23 May 1978.

7. Leah Margulies, 'Exporting infant malnutrition', *Health Right*, Vol. III, 2, 1977.

8. London, 1974.

Index